Food, Feelings and Freedom:
The End to Emotional Eating

Food, Feelings and Freedom:
The End to Emotional Eating

By Amber Stevens
LMT, CINHC

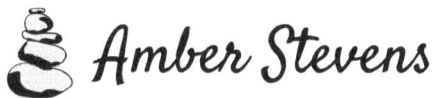

Amber Stevens

Amber Stevens, LLC
2019

2019
978-0-578-59350-0
Amber Stevens, LLC
Arvada, CO 80002
www.YouAreBoundless.com

About
The Author

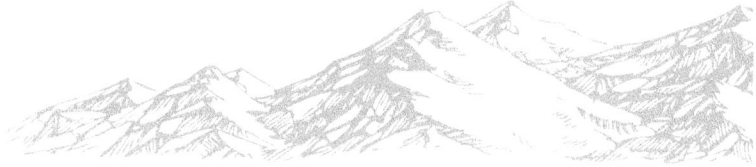

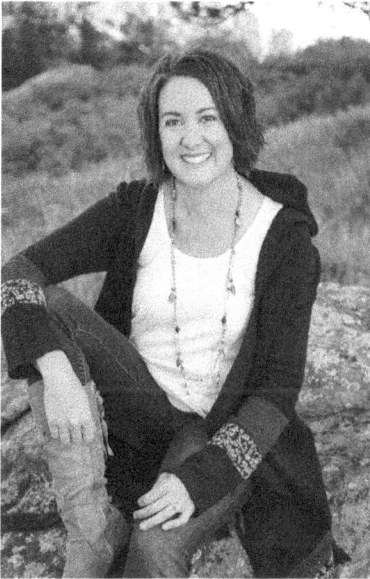

Amber Stevens is an Integrative Nutrition Health Coach, Mindful Based Eating (MB-Eat) Coach, and a Licensed Massage Therapist.

Passionate about helping people to connect with their bodies in a loving and supportive way as well as holding a B.A. in Technical Journalism, she has married her love of nutrition and healthy living with writing to bring this book to life.

Amber is the mother of two amazing boys, wife to the greatest man alive, and owner/operator of Amber Stevens, LLC.

You can learn more about Amber at **www.YouAreBoundless.com**

For fun advice and tips on mindful eating and living, follow her on Facebook **@FoodPositive**

Sign up for the newsletter at **www.YouAreBoundless.com**

Contents

Welcome

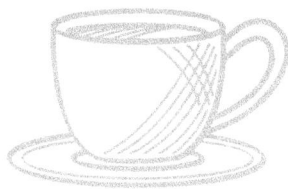

Hello there!

If you are reading this book, it means that you are ready to be back in the driver's seat of your life. You recognize that emotions have power, and they like to throw their weight around like a rambunctious toddler. But I'm here to tell you that **you** are in charge. You have control over your emotions, and you can put those emotions in time out!

This book isn't about enforcing hard rules. It's about understanding and self-compassion. It's a loving approach to gaining awareness about your personal habits of emotional eating and feeling empowered to make the choices that support your overall well-being.

Information in this book is drawn from nutrition science, neuroscience, biology, anatomy, and life experiences. But I promise only to give you enough science and background information to answer the "what is happening to me?" question without weighing you down with an information overload.

Reading this book should be a stress-free endeavor. (Who needs more "to-dos" right?) Read it at your own pace - a chapter here and there or a paragraph before bed. Read straight through or skip around and jump ahead to chapters that resonate with you in the moment. You are reading this because you want change. **You want more joy and less pain.** This is the information you need. But while this book will help with insight, easy to follow steps, and food recommendations, it is **you** that affects change. Make the commitment to yourself to support your body and health with love and gentleness. Give yourself permission to put yourself first at this time, and let my words act as your guide.

This is your journey, so move at a pace that allows you to connect with yourself and prepare your mind, body, and heart for an end to emotional eating.

The Journey
Why I Wrote This

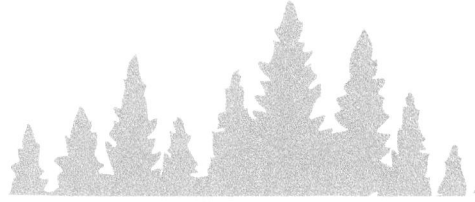

When I consider why I wrote Food, Feelings and Freedom, I realize that it all boils down to one major reason: We are all amazing, beautiful people, and it's about time that we realize it. No, not just realize it - Live it!

My journey with emotional eating starts in my childhood. I'll share some of my early experiences with food throughout the book, but for now, you should know that I watched my mom struggle with her weight and health for my whole life (and most of hers). When I was young, I didn't know that she was obese; I knew I loved my mommy. And while she struggled with her weight, she never once made me think about my own weight. I thank her for that - growing up is tough enough without body issues.

At fourteen, after a series of lethargy and fainting spells, I was diagnosed with hypoglycemia, or low blood sugar. My doctor told me to avoid sugar, or, "If you're going to eat it, have it with protein." The only protein I was aware of was cheese and meat. So I continued to drink my 32 ounce Dr. Pepper and eat my chocolate malted ice cream and my Three Musketeers… with a cheeseburger.

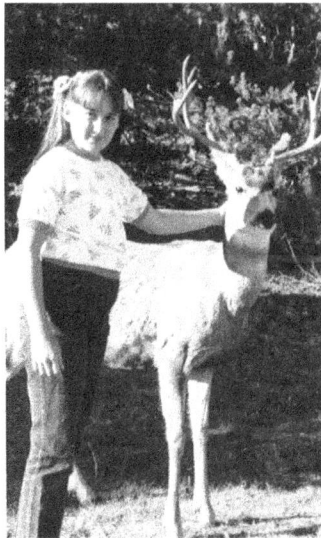

Somehow, at sixteen, I lost a ton of weight. Good metabolism and a bunch of after-school activities kept me tall, thin, and dorky. But I lost so much weight over one summer that my school counselor questioned me about bulimia on more than one occasion. In one year, I went from barely being aware of my body to being hyperaware - and critical. I started to believe that I wasn't enough - pretty enough, good enough. I often became deeply depressed, so I often ate candy.

The Journey: Why I Wrote This

I was twenty-three when my world blew open, and I discovered there was a whole other world of strange fruits, vegetables, and something called "organic" foods. My husband taught me that tuna came in steaks not cans!

This is when I started noticing **what** people eat, what I eat. But for years, I paid attention only to the "data of food" - carbs, calories, protein, and more. I focused on nutrition information and thought it was all anyone needed to know.

Then my mom went through the Lap Band procedure to shrink her belly and lose weight. Someday I may write about her (our) story with this, but for now, here's a quick summary of what happened: Mom lost the weight; Mom still ate unhealthily; Mom's doctor wanted to prescribe her with an antidepressant...an *antidepressant*!

Whoa! What?! My mom is a happy person. She does **not** need antidepressants. That was the moment that I realized how poorly she had been eating and how food could help her to stay off the medications.

> **"**
>
> **This experience lead me to start noticing how people eat, and how I eat. I realized that food was just the start. The mind has a strong opinion on what nutrients the body needs. It isn't the stomach lacking food; it is the mind lacking food!**
>
> **"**

My experience of being raised in a "dieting" home made me strive to lead a better, healthier life. And I did that. I maintained a healthy weight (with some fluctuations here and there). I had all the nutrition data. I earned my certificates. I worked with hundreds of clients. Yet, I missed my own connection with my emotions. See I was always the strong and stable one growing up. And for a long time, I worked in male-dominated environments. Emotions were not allowed.

And then my kids came along. I was busy before, but this was a whole new level of "mom-busy." I pushed my emotions down, down, down. I was in control, right?

Then the panic attacks started... and fainting. I saw doctors, certain that I had, at worst, a tumor or, at best, an unhealthy relationship with gravity.

The doctors couldn't provide answers but diagnosed me with Vasovagal syncope. This is a fancy way to say that my vagus nerve over (or under) reacts and then I faint (syncope).

When I began researching the vagus nerve, there it was. Stress. This nerve is largely influenced by stress. So I took stock of my life. I looked in the mirror - **really looked**. Staring back at me was not brown hair and annoying chin whiskers *(thanks grandma)* but pain, anger, disappointment, worry, and fear.

All the emotions that I had pushed away, believing that I was doing myself a favor.

I paused and reflected (it is a mirror after all). *How did I get here?* I wondered. *I'm the healthy one. I'm the one who knows what and how to do it.*

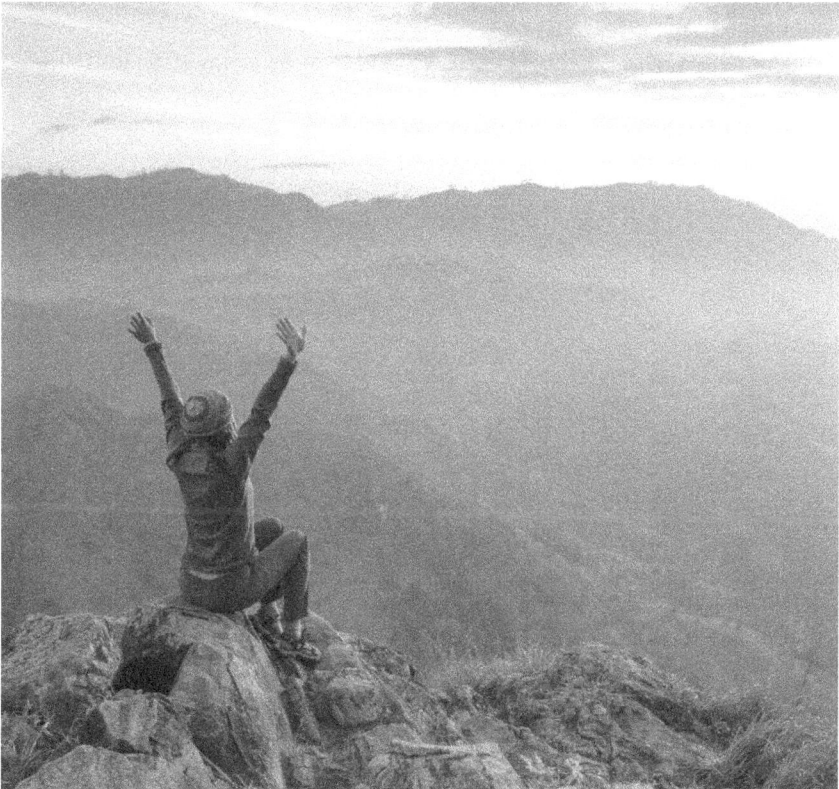

The Journey: Why I Wrote This

So I started to pay attention and was amazed at what I learned:

I was eating bags of chocolate at work because it gave me a sense of control whenever I felt overwhelmed.

I was eating ice cream before bed because that is what I craved with my second son and it comforted me.

I craved cheese and potato chips because fat and salt were delicious and they reminded me of home, of love.

I was eating fast and mindlessly.

*I was gaining weight and I was **not** healthy.*

I made a decision. This was not the real me. This was an imposter, and she was no longer allowed to take residence in my body!

I took several steps to change, which have transformed my life. I still have emotions *(thankfully)*. I still have cravings. But I know what to do. I know what my body is really saying it needs. I know that I am the **real** me and I feel **great** in my body!

Ready to take these steps? Then keep reading and start today!

Why Do We Eat When
Our Emotions
Kick In?

Emotions are amazing and part of what make us human. We can laugh, cry, yearn, scream, or feel all warm and fuzzy at times. Emotions help to give us personality and charisma. But there can be a dark side to emotions; a side that makes us feel out of control in our lives. This dark side seems to make our choices for us even before we are completely aware of what's happening.

This is especially true for emotional eaters. Do you find that you automatically grab a certain food at the same time each day? When you are sad or bored, do you look for answers in the cabinets or the refrigerator? Has ice cream become your best friend after a long, stressful day? If you answered yes to any of these questions, you are not alone... not even close. The mom in the car in front of you is eating cookies as she drives. The co-worker next to you has M&M's in her drawer. The truth is we all eat for emotional comfort at times.

The problem exists, however, when we always turn to food for comfort, causing us to eat more calories than we need, often with little nutritional value. The problem deepens, then, with how we feel about ourselves after eating these foods. We often feel like a failure. As if we did not live up to some expectation of ourselves - an expectation that we likely haven't even identified.

This then creates a vicious circle, and we turn to food to comfort our feelings of inadequacy. This is the problem. We eat. We don't want to eat. We want to eat. We feel ashamed for eating. We eat again. We look in the mirror and ask, "Why can't I stop? What is wrong with me?"

Does this sound like you? Maybe it's not so bad. You are aware that you eat emotionally, but you're still feeling pretty healthy. You just want to be and do better.

But maybe it is bad. You are gaining weight. You are feeling depressed and trying to hide from the world, from yourself.

Regardless of your level of emotional eating, there are simple solutions. Before we get into those, let's first take a closer look at the problem. Why does food soothe us?

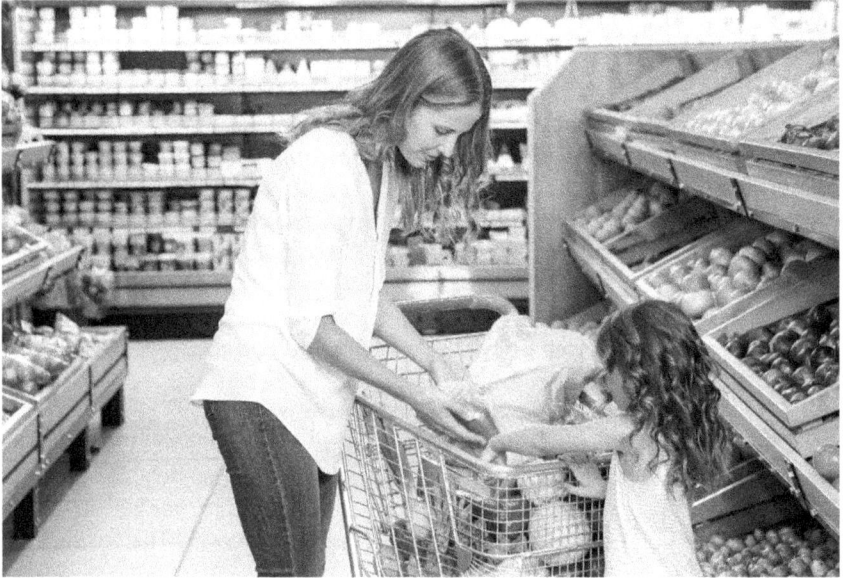

⊙ For Starters - It's a Learned Behavior.

You learned the behavior of emotional eating a long time ago, most likely as a child. If you're old enough to remember the 1980's PSA against drugs, there's a classic moment where the kid yells, "I learned it from watching you dad!" Nearly 40 years later, this has become a bit of a joke, but it still holds truth. As children, we learned our behaviors by watching others, especially our parents.

When your mom was sad, did she bake cookies with you and eat them until they were gone? Did your dad take out his stress and anger on a bag of potato chips? Was sugar a go-to in your home when tensions rose? This is all pretty standard. But you watched and repeated, subconsciously learning how to deal with your emotions by turning to food.

Research shows that by the time you were seven years old, your core circuits were built. Anything that made you feel good built pathways to your "happy chemicals" (we'll talk about those in a moment), telling you, "This is good for me!" Likewise, whatever felt bad built pathways to tell your brain and your body, "This is bad for me." Seven is young, but how often was food offered as a reward when you were a child? You behaved well at school - ice cream time! You stopped throwing a tantrum - here's a cookie! We learn to associate food and reward very early in life.

But we don't stop growing or learning at seven, so there are plenty of opportunities to learn new behaviors and further establish these core circuits. You continued to watch your parents and your friends for confirmation of what to do and how to do it.

There were also those moments growing up where you didn't know what to do. I know as a teenager you thought you knew it all - we all did - but we were always looking for answers. Sometimes, our parents or another adult wasn't someone we wanted to turn to. That's the moment that food became a close friend. It wouldn't tell your secrets. Food wasn't going to judge you. Food was there - and always available - to help comfort and to bring joy (even if only for a moment). Somewhere you learned to eat in your room after bedtime. You learned to keep candy bars in your backpack at school. You learned that sugary and fatty foods made you feel better.

For example, when I was growing up, my bus stop was in front of a 7/11 convenience store. Almost daily, I would get off the bus, go into the store, and buy either a 32 oz Dr. Pepper and a Three Musketeers candy bar or a malted ice cream. Sometimes I would be crazy and buy all three! I learned to look forward to the end of the school day. I learned that there was a "good feeling" coming in just a few short hours. Then of course my blood sugar would crash before dinner, and I felt terrible. But that never stopped me. Why? Because my emotions wanted what they wanted, and I had not yet learned that I was actually the one in charge.

◉ Food Becomes a Reward

We also learned that food was a wonderful reward. Growing up, my family didn't spend money freely. We had the essentials. I got a new My Little Pony every Christmas, and we bought new clothes before school started. But when something was great or went particularly well, we went out to eat! While sometimes this was simply a trip to Sonic or Big Burger World, this was always a reward. On truly special reward days, we went to a Mexican restaurant called Chili Wagon. They had the best bean burrito dripping in melted cheese!

On those days, I felt rewarded. I felt that I was being good (a good daughter, a good student, a good weed puller...) simply because we ate out instead of in. And my mom was an excellent cook, so I didn't feel deprived at home. I just connected "special restaurant food" with the emotion of pride.

Now, as an adult, I know that when I am feeling down on myself I automatically want to eat out. Restaurants put me in a good mood because they pull on my childhood heartstrings and tell me: "See, you are doing good. You are a good person!"

Amazing what our emotional connections to food can do for us!

As a child, I also learned the "Sneak Reward." This was one of my dad's favorite rewards. Notice I said "sneak" and not "surprise." I didn't come home one day and Dad yelled "Surprise!" and handed me a chocolate chip cookie. No, the Sneak Reward showed up during my mom's ongoing dieting attempts.

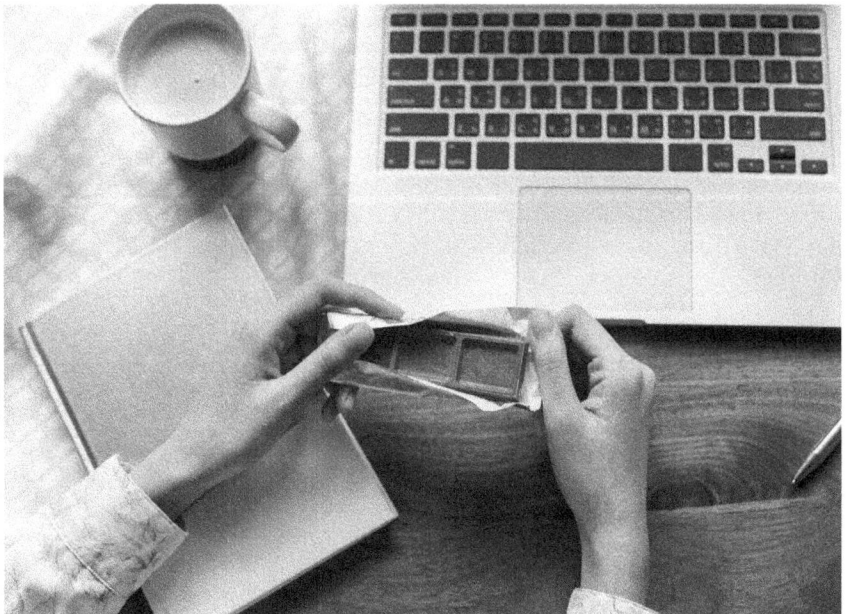

During several months when we had dined on salads (usually iceberg lettuce versions), soups (think broths), and were about to be introduced to the cabbage soup diet, Dad picked me up at school one day and said, "Let's have lunch." Now that was a reward in itself, but it got better. We were going out for burgers! Now I already covered that eating out was a big deal for me, but adding cheeseburgers to the mix after many cold salads was amazing! And it was for Dad too. But we had to sneak it: "Shhhh. Don't tell your mother."

I learned in this moment the bliss of reward and the shame of guilt. (We'll talk about the shame/guilt cycle later in this chapter. This is an important cycle to acknowledge, especially if it goes unchecked.)

When you look at your eating habits, can you identify the moment that you learned them? Who was there? What were you feeling? Have you continued to turn to food when those same feelings arise? This is normal.

I'm glad you're here, reading this book, because there is a solution. But there is more to the problem than just learned behaviors and rewards.

Hormones - More Accurately - Chemicals

It's the "H" word: hormones. I think it's both a blessing and a curse to know about our hormones. It's a blessing because we have insight into what is driving or motivating our choices, especially around and about food. It's a curse, because it can be challenging to overcome our hormonal surges even when we are intimately familiar with them.

It may be a surprise to learn that our motivations and reactions are not solely fueled by hormones however. There are strong chemicals, called neurotransmitters that affect them. You've likely heard of the most famous one - **dopamine**.

Neurotransmitters and hormones are two types of chemical signaling that allow communication to flow through the body. Neurotransmitters are the molecules used by the nervous system to transmit messages between neurons or from neurons to muscles.(1) It's like giving the person next to you a high five. Hormones, however, are released into the bloodstream to reach targets anywhere in the body.(2) This is communication more in line with sending a text or posting on social media. Both communication styles influence your emotional responses - fast or slow, intense or weak, frequent or short-lived.

Since knowledge is power, let's reveal the systems at play with our emotions. As promised, this book does not deep dive into science, so I'm only presenting what you need to know about hormones and neurotransmitters. I'll mention these throughout the book (especially the first four), so take a moment to get familiar with them but don't feel like you need to hurt your brain!

"

I think it's both a blessing and a curse to know about our hormones. It's a blessing because we have insight into what is driving or motivating our choices, especially around and about food. It's a curse, because it can be challenging to overcome our hormonal surges even when we are intimately familiar with them.

"

Introducing the Four Primary "Happiness" Chemicals: dopamine, serotonin, oxytocin and endorphin.(3)

Dopamine - the "reward" neurotransmitter. Dopamine produces joy from finding things that meet your need; it's the "I got it!" feeling.

Serotonin - the "pride" neurotransmitter. Serotonin creates a feeling of being respected by others; it's the "good job!" feeling.

Oxytocin - the "bonding" neurotransmitter. Oxytocin produces a feeling of being safe with others or a good feeling from having social alliances.

Endorphin - produces euphoria. Endorphins mask pain, primarily physical pain.

⊙ Other Key Players

Estrogen - a hormone that influences your mood through neurotransmitters. Estrogen can increase serotonin, dopamine, and endorphins, creating positive mood states. Low estrogen levels are associated with depression and mood swings. However, high estrogen can create a sense of tension, anxiety, and irritability.

Progesterone - another hormone which balances (or should balance) estrogen levels in the body. Where estrogen is excitatory, progesterone is calming. An imbalance between these two hormones can cause anxiety and sleep issues. Progesterone calms the brain by activating gamma-aminobutyric acid (GABA) receptors.

GABA - an inhibitory neurotransmitter that slows down the activity of the limbic system (the emotional control center in the brain) reducing fear, anxiety, and panic.

Acetylcholine (ACH) - the primary neurotransmitter in charge of muscle movement, alertness, concentration, and memory. When ACH is optimal, you are in a good mood and your mind is clear and focused. ACH and serotonin work together in an inverse relationship - one goes up, the other goes down. Since ACH controls primitive drives and emotions, like anger and fear, too much of it can cause depression and anger.

Cortisol - your body's primary stress hormone, also known as the "fight or flight" hormone. Cortisol is a powerful and necessary hormone for survival, but when it is out of balance, it wreaks havoc on your body and your emotions. Specific to the female brain, cortisol blocks oxytocin, shutting off the desire for affection.[4] You'll learn about cortisol in the next chapter as I highlight its connection to stress.

Epinephrine/norepinephrine - more commonly known as adrenalin and noradrenalin, and both act as hormones and neurotransmitters in your body. Both are released during a flight or fight response to deal with blood pressure, heart rate, and glucose conversion. These contribute to a feeling of depression, anxiety, panic, fatigue, and nervousness. *Dopamine is converted into norepinephrine.*

Why Do We Eat When Our Emotions Kick In?

Our mood is largely regulated by **Monoaminergic systems** in our body. *(Memorize this word and see if you can slide it into conversation at a party!)* This system uses monoamine neurotransmitters to process and regulate emotions, arousal, and certain types of memory. Serotonin, epinephrine, and dopamine are all examples of these types of systems. All monoamines derive from amino acids - phenylalanine, tyrosine, and tryptophan to name a few famous ones. The foods recommended in this book are intended to affect the monoamines and the "mood systems" in our bodies.

So What Do These Chemicals Want From Us?

Overall the brain wants to be free from danger (i.e. pain) and rewarded for its great job of surviving. Or, another day alive - let's eat!

But since pain exists and real or perceived dangers surround us daily (or hourly), our brain and our body seeks ways to stop the pain and discomfort and keep going. This is called coping.

Coping

Coping is the ability to deal effectively with something difficult (or so says the dictionary). At best, it means to look after yourself. At worst, it means to survive, to keep your head above water, and not drown. I've personally felt both scenarios.

But what are we really coping from? Was traffic truly so terrible? Was shrinking your favorite sweater really a disaster? Was listening to children crying the end of the world? No. While it feels like a yes sometimes, in the big picture, it really isn't something that we have to "survive."

What we are actually coping with is our own inner voice. The voice that judges and critiques our every move and decision. It is the voice of the **Inner Critic**, and it is quick to tell us how poorly we are doing as a human being.

Your inner critic tells you, "Your child is still crying. You are a terrible mother for not finding a way to have better behaved children." Your inner critic tells you, "Your pants are too tight. You are too weak to stick to a diet. You should just give up and stop trying to be something you are not - skinny."

Your inner critic tells you, "You are going to miss that deadline at work. Everyone knows you aren't that good at your job. You're a phony."

The critic is loud and repetitive. The broken record spins, and some time long ago you learned that **a certain food quieted the voice**. A favorite food - chocolate, cake, cheese, pizza, chips - helped you to cope and even to ignore the inner critic.

But coping is the only solution you have found because the voice never goes away. The voice is you. The voice is the record you made for yourself while you were growing up. It is triggered whenever a situation arises that makes you **feel** like you did when it was first created.

When you were yelled at as a child, you were hurt and scared, and a voice appeared. It told you that you weren't doing right and not to do that again. (Maybe you forgot to put away the milk.) When you're yelled at as an adult, you're hurt and scared, and the same voice reminds you not to do that again. (Maybe you crashed the car.)

Different situation but same emotion equals the same voice.

Surprisingly, the voice exists to protect you. It is trying to help. It wants only to keep you safe. Since you created the voice, you can change it. You can learn new ways to comfort and soothe yourself. You will learn how in this book.

The Guilt and Shame Cycle

Remember the cheeseburger reward from my dad? The one that I couldn't tell my mom about? I mentioned that I felt guilty, as if I had committed some burger crime in the food mafia. This was, of course, my own perception. No crime was committed, but I felt ashamed for wanting the burger.

In my wellness practice, I have come to recognize two types of guilt and shame: (1)actual and (2) perceived. These may seem obvious, but let's examine them in a bit more detail.

Actual guilt occurs when you know what you are doing is wrong, but do it anyway. You feel guilty and ashamed but, in most cases, can't change what you did. In this case, food eases the pain that comes from having wronged someone else. Food offers quiet support when you feel that you cannot share what happened with others. Food gives a false sense that "everything is OK" (especially when sugar is involved).

Perceived guilt occurs when you torment yourself with the "I should be" or "I used to be" conversation. The conversation looks a bit like the following:

- *"I should be 30 pounds lighter by now. I just can't stick to a diet, but I do try. Then it all goes wrong again."*
- *"I used to be a size 4! Now I'm a 16. I just can't eat like I used to, but I love pizza so much."*
- *"I should be putting the kids in music lessons. They really need to learn an instrument to go to college."*
- *"I used to run marathons. I don't understand why I'm so slow. I'm just lazy now I guess."*

Your perceptions of yourself sets you up for success or failure, for reward or shame. If you consistently compare your 40 year-old self with your 20 year-old self, you will likely be let down. (At least physically speaking; I'm so much wiser now!)

If you focus on the "used to," then you are not focusing on the amazing possibilities in the "I am!" Likewise, if you focus on the "should be," you miss out on the "right now!" You miss the beauty that is in you in this present moment.

In both cases, you create a situation primed for judgement. How do you judge yourself? Did you decide that you failed because you **feel** you should be 30 pounds lighter and now you feel guilty for not meeting that expectation? And now you feel ashamed for letting yourself "get this way?" And now you eat.

You eat mindlessly - simply eating more for the purpose of feeling better. But you are trying to feel better about feeling ashamed for not losing weight, and now you feel guilty again for eating. So the cycle continues.

Food can and does provide comfort. But it does not break the cycle. It acts as a soothing companion as you bounce around in the guilt and shame spin cycle. But you can break this cycle - the steps provided in this book will provide you with some methods of how you can start to break it. And once the cycle is broken you can feel the freedom from your emotional eating, living with confidence and self-respect!

⊙ Looking to the Outside

Emotions cause another problem in our lives: they cause us to seek solutions and ways to cope that are external to our actual needs.

When guilt and other emotions are specifically related to losing weight, we turn to diet plans. Books and videos on weight loss are a multibillion dollar industry that target our emotions because it's our feelings that motivate us

Why Do We Eat When Our Emotions Kick In?

to eat. Whether we actually feel hungry or just sad, we eat!

But most diets come and go without lasting benefits. These are the Fad Diets - the "quick fixes" that promise to make everything OK. And maybe they do - but only for a short period of time, because often these diets are Restriction Diets masquerading as Lifestyle Changes.

Restriction diets are methods of eating that require you to eliminate foods (cheese or wheat) or even whole food groups (dairy or carbs). Restriction diets are difficult to sustain because you are creating strict rules around your food and eating habits.

Rules are hard to maintain in ever changing circumstances, and you feel the gnawing desire that "just a little is fine" growing as the days go by. You do not live in a vacuum; avoiding sugar at home may be easy, but avoiding it at the company holiday party may not be.

When you give in to "just a little won't hurt," but then eat more than just a little, you open the doors to guilt. That guilty voice says, "Well, now you blew it. You might as well keep eating." This is known as the **Abstinence-Violation (AV) Effect**(5) (yep, science has a term for "blowing it"). The A/V Effect can strike at any time and is a feeling that keeps us from meeting new goals. But good news - now you know what it is, so you can do something about it. And some solutions are at your fingertips in this book!

When our emotions arise, we often look outward towards food. It's so easy and readily available, coming in all shapes and sizes, and we don't even have to get out of our car to get food. Sugar and fatty foods are the "emotional eating all-stars" and are the foods we turn to most for support.

There are three simple reasons for this:

1. *Sugar and fat were scarce in the wild, so biologically, we have adapted to release dopamine and serotonin in the brain which makes us feel good and happy and encourages us to seek out more of these foods. It's basic survival!*
2. *Sugar reduces cortisol, releasing stressful feelings.*
3. *Fat and sugar feed the brain! You think, therefore you eat!*

Whatever your food of choice (and perhaps your preferred food is "whatever is available"), reaching for food to cope with your feelings is a short-term solution. You have not changed the circumstances that caused your off feeling; you simply covered it up.

Remember, food isn't always the solution we seek. Shopping can offer the same benefit dopamine can. You went looking for something, found it, and your brain says "Way to go!" You feel better buying things, but again, you have not fixed the issue that urged you to go shopping in the first place.

Shopping isn't always a negative thing. It's only a problem when your bank account can't support it, or when you have to cut a path through your bedroom to sleep at night! And the same goes for food. So just as buying things you don't need, or even really want, is a signal that you are in a coping mode, so is eating food you don't need or even really want. And both show that you are really seeking solutions to heal your emotions.

Let's start the healing now!

Emotions vs. Feelings

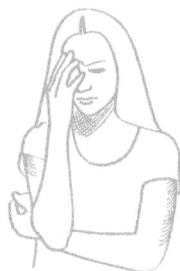

I've introduced you to the problems and concerns with emotional eating, along with the chemical cocktail that arouses your brain to desire certain moods. Now let's take a closer look at how your brain interprets input from these chemicals and life experiences to create an emotion.

Emotions and feelings are not the same thing. Strange. We use the words interchangeably, but they are actually quite distinct.

Emotions are a **physical response in the body**. Something has engaged our brain and our senses in such a manner as to cause a release of hormones and neurotransmitters which provides input to our brain.

What does the brain then do with that input? It interprets it. It makes millisecond decisions about what to do and how to do it. Sometimes this is immediate and out of our control, like stepping on a nail and jerking your foot upward. This is clearly a good thing.

Sometimes, this is quick with little conscious awareness on our part. Imagine that you were suddenly facing a bear in your path. Neurotransmitters would send a message: "Hey this is dangerous!" The brain would quickly recognize an immediate threat and send the message to your feet to run like the wind. Or if you have backcountry wilderness experience, it would tell you to stand tall and back away while making a noisy racket.

Sometimes, the interpretation is slower, allowing the brain to key in to many areas to support its decision in what to do next. This is called assessing.

The brain assesses the danger potential of each moment based on existing experience and knowledge. **It relies on patterns to make decisions**. Hold this thought in your mind for a moment as we'll come back to it.

Feelings on the other hand are **psychological constructs of the mind**. We create our own feelings. Which is great news! Since you created your feelings, you can control them!

But it also means that your experience of feeling a certain way is unique to you. When you get angry, you may stomp around the house and yell at everyone. Your friend, however, gets angry and "anger cleans" her whole house, not even speaking a word to anyone!

American psychologist, Dr. Robert Plutchik has identified 34,000 distinguishable emotions, yet he has proposed that there are actually only eight primary emotions that drive our feelings. These are joy, sadness, acceptance, disgust, fear, anger, surprise, and anticipation.(7)

Does this surprise you? It certainly surprised me (but hey, that's one of the eight emotions), until I understood that emotions and feelings are different. Let's look at joy for example. You can have the emotion of joy" and feel happy, content, blissful, excited, pleased with yourself, proud, and more. These "feelings" are all synonyms to describe joy, but our brilliant minds have created characteristics for each of these feelings in our bodies.

When we have an emotion, our nerves have the same communication within our brains. For example, adrenaline is released into the body, creating an emotional reaction such as fear (which causes cortisol to release, but we'll discuss that more later). Our hands sweat, our breath shortens. This is largely the same from person to person.

But when we have a feeling, it is not the same every time. When we feel happy, it is not the same as when we feel excited. You don't wear the same smile or walk the same way. With happy, you may walk peacefully through your day and buy a coffee for the stranger behind you. With excitement, you may be calling everyone you know, bouncing down the street, and talking super fast about your amazing thing. Your responses to your feelings are different than your neighbors', family's, and friends' responses.

Now, let's go back to assessment and pattern recognition. When you first felt an emotion (a chemical release), all of your senses (humans have far more than just the big five(6)) sent information to the brain; what you were touching and its texture and temperature, what you were tasting, what you were smelling, where you were in the room, where you were in the world, the colors you saw, and so much more. From all of this data your mind (a creating machine) created a **feeling** for you to associate with that emotion. Now each time your body has that same chemical cocktail, you feel that same feeling.

This is why our feelings are so personal. Have you told someone, "You just don't understand!" Well, true. They don't know your exact feeling, but they most likely understand the emotion.

With this knowledge, take a look at your patterns with your feelings.

Do you eat chocolate when you are sad? Do you eat pastries (simple carbs) when you are frustrated? Do you eat "anything sugar" when you are bored?

Whatever it may be, this is your pattern. This is how you've handled your feelings after your body has an emotion. And since it's your pattern, the brain will go to it every single time you have that emotion. Every. Single. Time.

Remember, I said, "The brain assesses the danger potential of each moment based on existing experience and knowledge." If anger is a threat (which it is in our brain's way of thinking), then based off previous experiences of what helped before (tearing through a bag of chips) it will **strongly** suggest that you take the same action and **now** to get better.

While we can't necessarily change the flood of chemicals that give us emotions, we **can** change the way we feel about them!

▶ What Chemicals Create Emotions

Remember the "happiness" chemicals? They are dopamine, serotonin, oxytocin, and endorphins. These are the top four when it comes to feeling happy or sad, elated or depressed, at ease or in pain. As you read in the previous chapter, they work along with many other chemicals to create the desired (or undesired) emotion.

However, I want to call out three specific chemicals a little bit deeper here: the neurotransmitters dopamine and serotonin and the hormone cortisol.

Since dopamine is tied to our reward system, it comes into play during most emotional states. I'm calling it the "Goldilocks" hormone: too much and you can develop an addiction; too little and you become depressed; just the right amount, and you feel happy and satisfied.

Have you ever thought "I'm addicted to sugar?" I hear this one many times a day. You are not actually addicted to sugar. You are more likely addicted to the "feel good" feeling that you get when you eat sugar, which happens due to the surge in dopamine. Your body is rewarding you for eating something that was once hard to find in nature.

> **You are not actually addicted to sugar. You are more likely addicted to the "feel good" feeling that you get when you eat sugar, which happens due to the surge in dopamine.**

The only problem here is that when you become addicted to the "feel good" state, you tend to eat sugar to feel that way again and again. The dopamine receptors build up an immunity to sugar *(like iocane powder... you're welcome Princess Bride fans)*, and then you need more and more sugar to get the same release of dopamine as you did before. You stop eating sugar once your body rewards you!

If you don't believe me, try this simple test: fill a cup with ¼ cup of table sugar and eat it.

What? That doesn't appeal to you? You can't possibly eat that much sugar? But this is close to the amount of sugar in a 22 ounce soda!

Most of us can easily drink a 22 ounce soda, so why can't we eat the ¼ cup of sugar? Because we are **not** addicted to sugar. We are addicted to the dopamine high, but we have enough self-control to choose the method in which that sugar is delivered.

⊙ Sugar Cravings

Our bodies need sugar. It is the prefered fuel source for our body. Our brain alone uses about 20% of glucose-derived energy, but it only accounts for less than 2% of body weight!(8) Glucose metabolism (creating energy from sugar) provides for the generation of neurotransmitters and for physiological brain functions (among other things).

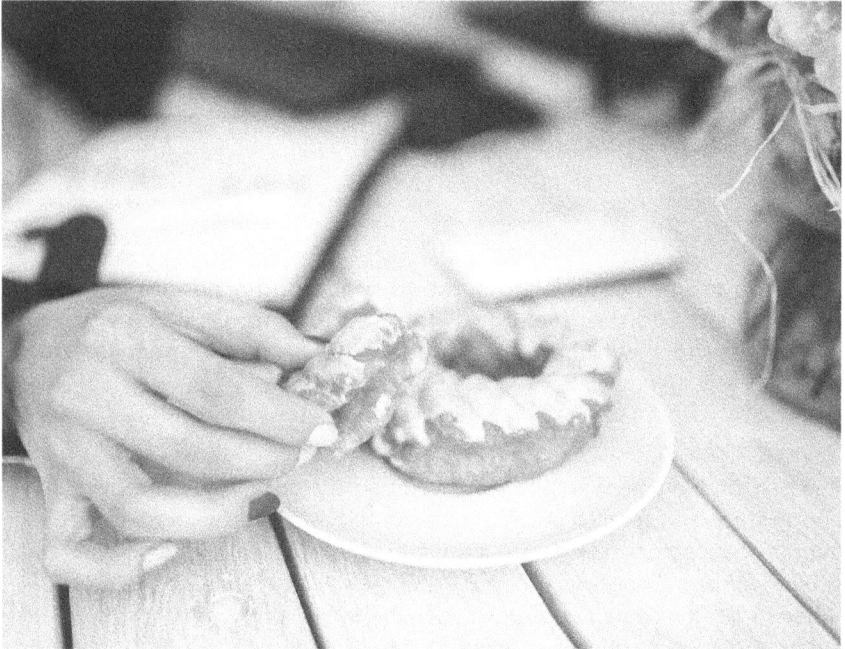

While we need it, it's important to understand that not all sugars are created equal. Food contains glucose, fructose, lactose, sucrose, and more. This book isn't a full lesson on sugar varieties, but I mention it here because sugar, overall, has a bad rap, and I want you to feel informed and empowered in your diet, especially when it involves sugar.

Glucose vs. Fructose vs. Sucrose

When you crave sugar, what are you actually craving? This is unique to everyone, because sugar comes in many forms. Most people think they are craving the pure "white" stuff, or table sugar. This is sucrose.

But sucrose is equal parts **glucose** and **fructose** and is also found naturally in fruits and vegetables.

Fructose and glucose are both simple sugars, meaning that they break down and burn quickly as energy. Fructose is mostly available in fruits, honey, and some vegetables. Glucose is often found in fruits, simple carbohydrates, and starches. Glucose is also in milk as part of lactose.

All sugars feed your body in various ways and perform certain tasks to keep cells functioning and energized. There are two reasons you crave sugar:

1. *You need more energy (glucose). Your body has burned through its available glucose stores, and you need to feed it some nutrients. This is the "blood sugar" crash!*

2. *Your brain wants you to survive (fructose and glucose)!*

Blood sugar refers to the amount of glucose in your blood. Glucose is directly linked to how much we eat. If glucose drops, our brain is signaled to eat more food (this is hunger). If glucose rises, it signals the brain that "you've eaten." Our body does this by using insulin to drive glucose into the cells. The glucose is either burned as energy or it is stored in the muscles and the liver as glycogen to use when needed *(when a bear chases you for example)*.

Often, a sugar craving strikes around 3pm. Why? Well, you need enough energy to get through your busy day. Energy comes from calories. The fastest way to get calories, and the easiest way to break down (digest) those calories, comes from sugar, specifically glucose.

If you always crave sugar in the afternoon, look back on your day and ask: did I eat a balanced breakfast? Did I eat a snack? Have I been running all day or sitting at a computer? Basically, did I meet my energy needs?

The other sugar, fructose is converted to glucose in the liver. If not needed, it is stored in the liver or as fat. When the body uses fructose, it does not use insulin. Without insulin secretion, your body never signals that "you've eaten." You do not get the cue to stop eating.*(9)* Fructose is needed to convert glycogen (stored glucose), however.

Also, fructose is shown to have a stronger impact on the reward center of the brain!*(10)* As you've learned, once upon a time calorie rich food was scarce and finding it was necessary for survival. Since fructose can be stored as fat, your brain has learned to reward you for eating high-fructose foods. Fat equals survival.

A high-fructose food can be fruit though. Rarely do people grab an apple when they have a sugar craving! So what is going on here? Why do you grab a cookie or pastry when a craving hits?

⊙➔ Our Second Brain

Did you know that you have two brains? Well, not two "brain organs" but two thinking and communicating machines in your body? One is your brain, and the other is your gut. Have you ever responded to something on a "gut instinct" or thought, "I just have a gut feeling about this?"

The brain and gut communicate with each other, and this is called the "Gut-Brain Axis." They speak to each other along communication channels through your nervous, immune, and endocrine (hormonal) systems.(11) So who's doing the talking? Bacteria!

You have a thriving microbiome - a habitat of tiny microorganisms - that send signals to your brain. There are billions of bacteria, each with their own unique chemical language. Each gives its input on "how you're feeling" and what kind of mood you are in, and this input is speedily sent along the systems for verification and feedback. They send the signals using the same neurotransmitters: dopamine, serotonin and GABA - all of which have antidepressant characteristics and are a primary way that gut bacteria influence our moods!

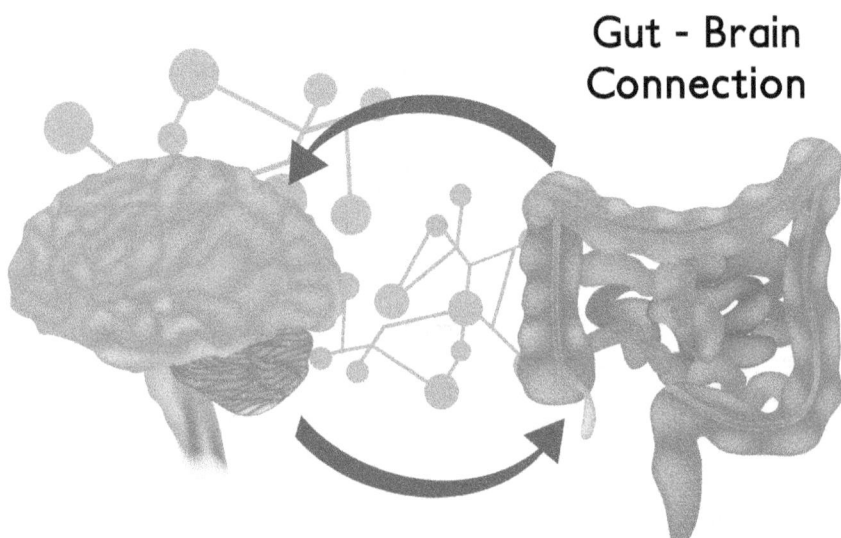

Gut - Brain Connection

What's more interesting is that 95% of serotonin is produced in the gut! We are not mentally aware of the serotonin in our gut. We don't say, "Oh, I can't eat very much today because I have too much serotonin this morning!" But we do respond to the serotonin because of the Gut-Brain Axis.

The brain and the bacteria are very similar in one trait - they both care about survival! Bacteria send these "feel good" hormones based on what you are eating, and whether or not **that food feeds them**. If you eat a doughnut, then that feeds the sugar-hungry bacteria (such as streptococcus) and it releases dopamine. Your brain registers the dopamine, and soon, you associate doughnuts with feeling good and you now crave doughnuts. The more you crave sugar, and eat it, the more **that specific bacteria** survives. (12)

So it's not really so much that you **are** what you eat, but rather that you **feel** what you eat.

Just like our bodies, the microbiota try to maintain homeostasis. **Depending on what you eat, you encourage different bacterial species to prosper. Variety is key here!** Each type of bacteria has its own food preferences. Bacteroidetes enjoy fat, Prevotella likes carbs and Bifido loves fiber. If you eat more fiber (feeding Bifido), you'll find your mood improving, and over time, you'll crave more fiber that makes you feel good!(13)

If you eat the same foods over and over (pizza and sweets), you feed the same bacteria. They thrive, taking over the "gut landscape" and demanding more of the same food. But if you eat different foods, then a huge diversity of bacteria can thrive, and they will work to balance each other out. Put another way - they will balance out your mood!

"

But if you eat different foods …. they will balance out your mood!

"

There is a great deal of research underway on the microbiome and the influence of food on our overall health. While I'm not going into depth on your second brain, it's important to give you a brief understanding that it exists and that food is absolutely connected to your emotional eating. Being aware that tiny organisms are saying "Feed me," should give you some power to say, "No! I'm not feeding you that!"

An out-of-balance microbiome also influences your cortisol levels, therefore stressing your body. But cortisol also influences a messy microbiome. Let's look at what this means for emotional eating.

The Stress Connection

Many people have written books on stress and for good reason - it wrecks us! Stress can have a good side, but its role in emotional eating is actually pretty dark. So let's shed some light on it.

Stress largely comes from the neurotransmitter adrenaline and the hormone cortisol. Cortisol kicks in when we are in a flight or fight state. The brain senses danger and we have to decide - stay and fight, get the heck out of there, or freeze and do nothing.

Cortisol is helpful to our bodies in that it:

- *Manages how the body uses carbohydrates, fats, and proteins,*
- *Increases blood sugar (glucose) to feed our cells and boost energy,*
- *Regulates the sleep/wake cycle,*
- *Regulates blood pressure, and*
- *Keeps inflammation down (yep that's correct - it's trying to help us!).*(14)

But when we have it in excess or it is uncontrolled in our bodies, cortisol is harmful, leading to a number of problems, including:

- *Anxiety and depression,*
- *Headaches and concentration problems,*
- *Digestive problems,*
- *Trouble sleeping, and*
- *Weight gain… just to name a few.*

During acute stress, or moments of temporary stress, cortisol helps you to manage the situation by getting the blood flowing to critical organs and muscles and motivating you towards resolution. During chronic stress however, the feedback loop that is supposed to control cortisol fails and the brain (and body) remains hyperactive. One specific area of the brain - the prefrontal cortex - is involved in higher thinking and executive control and regulation of emotions, impulses, desires, and cravings. Under stress, the prefrontal cortex is dampened, and the brain begins to rely on "automatic" behaviors and reward-based eating. The stressed brain expresses both a strong drive to eat and also an impaired capacity to inhibit eating!(15)

That's bad enough, but let's look at cortisol's relationship with insulin, since sugar is a major craving as we discussed. Insulin and cortisol play opposite roles. Insulin seeks to decrease energy levels (less sugar in the blood) while cortisol seeks to increase energy levels (fight or flight response).(16) This means that you are more likely to seek out sugar and fat when under stress as compared to "normal" or low stress moments. People with high cortisol reactivity report greater snacking in response to daily stressors!

"

The stressed brain expresses both a strong drive to eat and also an impaired capacity to inhibit eating!

"

The Stress Threshold

Stress can be helpful. It certainly saved us as a species many times. Stress by itself, as a concept, is not dangerous or "bad." Chronic stress, as discussed, can be harmful to your health. So what is chronic stress? Do you have it?

Only you can answer that question. It's important to recognize that each person has a "Stress Bucket," and on that bucket there is a line. You can fill that bucket again and again, right up to that line and your body will handle the stress in the correct manner, turning on and off as designed.

But if you cross that line, if you fill that bucket too high, then you trigger a stress response that is overpowering to your system. Hopefully, this is short lived and a rare occurrence.

The main problem, however, happens when you keep crossing that line. Your body stays stuck in the "on" position, constantly trying to fight off the danger. Your body sends hormones and messages across the channels, desperately trying to calm the adrenaline and the cortisol, but you keep crossing the line. Eventually, the message is no longer received.

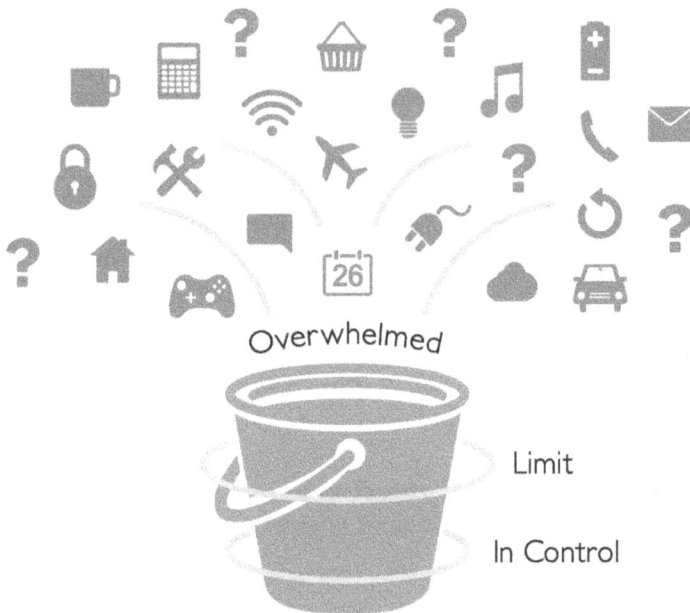

Overwhelmed

Limit

In Control

After time, the burden lowers the line on your bucket, so that even the smallest conflict or issue can set off the stress response. Your tolerance to stress is minimal, and life feels heavy.

So you turn to food. Food has been there for you, and it "magically" helps.

Stress causes you to eat out of balance or to overeat. It causes you to go on autopilot. Your brain has to deal with the threat (so don't bother it with other tasks), and your body just wants the easiest, and fastest, thing that will help return homeostasis. Food is simple. It's readily available. It's mindless.

Stress causes you to not eat at all. You are still on autopilot. Your brain has put such a high priority on eliminating the threat that it has shut down your body's need for anything else. Digestion is on hold, so food is out of the question.

Do you eat out of balance? Or do you skip your meals? Either way, your health suffers.

By overeating or eating unhealthy foods, you risk consuming far more calories than your body needs with most of those calories coming from high sugar and high fat sources. In moderation, these foods are great. In excess, they lead to weight gain, diabetes, cardiovascular disease, high blood pressure... The list is a long one.

By skipping food altogether, but especially during moments of high stress, you deprive your body of essential nutrients that it needs to restore balance to your body. You are further stressing your body by falsely adding to the brain's fear of danger. Your brain is thinking, "Ahhhhh we have no food," which pushes its focus deeper on the present stressor. If it can just get through this stressful moment, then all will be well.

So what are you to do? There's sugar everywhere, stress is a given, and now there's bacteria in your gut demanding food!

It's not hopeless - far from it. You are now fully aware of the problem and the driving forces behind your emotional eating. Knowing is half the battle! *(Who said that?...oh my, it was GI Joe! This book keeps getting more profound.)* And now that you know, you can do something about it!

Let's begin now with better food and lifestyle selections!

Foundational Solutions

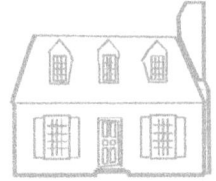

Before we dive into the best foods for moods, let's establish a solid foundation for success.

While diet and exercise are significant, you can consider them the walls and shell of the house. They hold everything together and make a pretty display, but if the house rests on shaky ground, it will crumble.

Below are some fundamental activities that you should practice regularly to support you with your emotional eating. These activities need to happen along with eating the right foods and moving your body. So let's address the fundamentals which are:

Sleep	*Massage*	*Aromatherapy*
Vitamin D	*Walking*	*Breathing*
Hydration	*Mindful Eating*	*Positive Mindset*

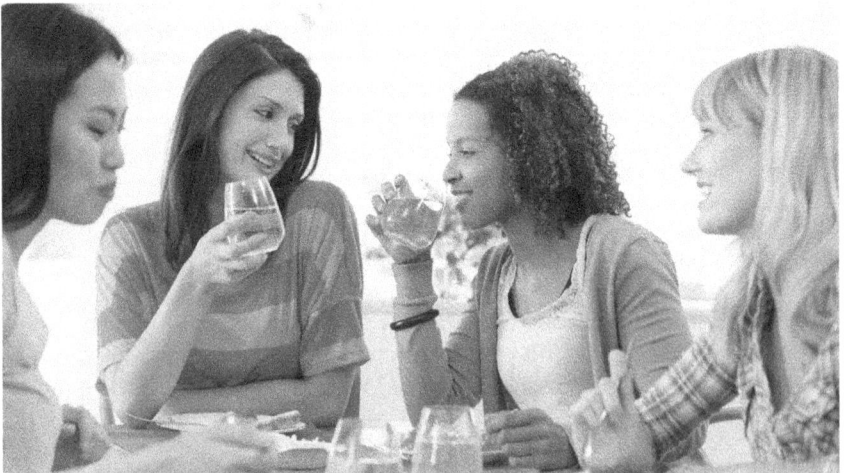

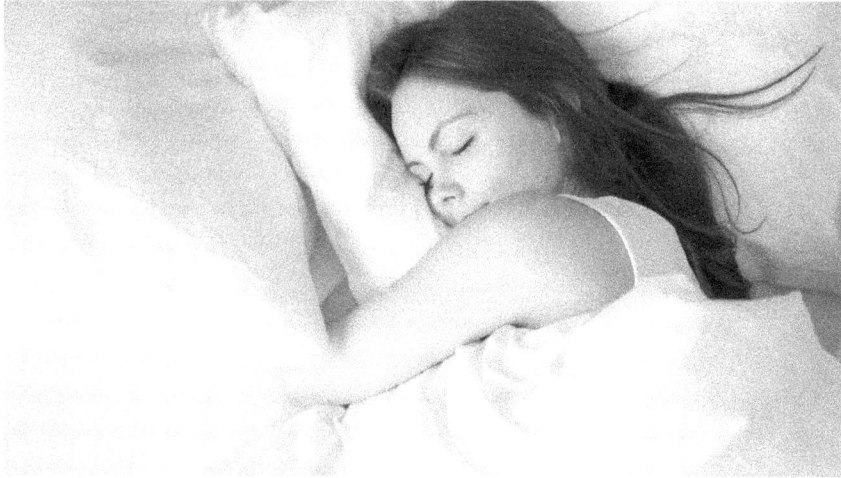

Sleep

I know that for many of you, sleep feels like a unicorn - a mythical creature that doesn't really exist, but we want so badly! This is exactly why sleep is the number one fundamental tool that you have to get right.

Sleep is responsible for repair and restoration of our bodies. It restores proper brain and physical health. It also keeps us in a functioning emotional state.(17) Sleep helps you to make decisions, be creative, pay attention, and cope with change. Not getting enough sleep (the amount that's right for you) may cause you to feel indecisive, depressed, angry, unable to cope, impulsive, and lacking in motivation. Physically, sleep deficiency is linked to an increased risk of heart and kidney disease, high blood pressure, obesity, and stroke (just to name a few).

Sleep and Emotional Stress

Numerous studies have shown a direct connection between quality of sleep, length of sleep, and emotions. If you are sleep deprived, you will tend to have less intense and less frequent positive moods (happiness for example) and are prone to have more intense and frequent negative moods (anger, fear, depression for example).

Sleep's effect on our emotions is a complicated one and is based on "time." Too little sleep or too much sleep can have a negative impact on your behavior. Likewise, sleep deprivation is a vicious cycle as sleep deprivation can compromise your ability to regulate your emotions, which then causes disrupted sleep, which further impairs your emotional well-being!(18)

So how do you know if you are getting enough sleep? For most of us, 7.5 to 8.5 hours of sleep is ideal. If you are getting less than that, consider your moods and energy levels during the day. If you are moody, hungry, fatigued, and "foggy" brained, there is a strong chance that you are sleep-deprived!

Sleep's Effect on Eating

You already know that "hunger" is your body's response to a drop in blood sugar in your cells. Well, sleep affects your body's reaction to insulin (the hormone that controls blood glucose). Sleep deficiency results in higher than normal blood sugar levels, which increases the risk of diabetes.

Sleep also helps with the "eating hormones" - ghrelin and leptin. Ghrelin makes you feel hungry, and leptin makes you feel full. When you are lacking in sleep, your level of ghrelin goes up and leptin goes down. Basically, you feel hungrier than if you had a good night's sleep!

Furthermore, our body burns fat while we sleep. Yep, you read that right - we lose weight in our sleep. But only with high quality sleep, the kind that deepens into the rapid eye movement (REM) state, and also only with a good duration of sleep (8.5 hours is ideal).(19) Most people manage to sleep only 5.5 hours, or even a little over 6 hours, but that loss of sleep causes a shift in metabolism which makes the body want to preserve fat (store energy) while also producing more of the appetite stimulating hormone ghrelin.

Ready? Let's Sleep More!

Now you are fully aware of how important sleep is in establishing healthy eating habits, a positive outlook, and overall physical and mental well-being. If your sleep pattern is out of whack (that is the scientific term), then here are some steps to better sleep:

Do not eat meals late at night.
Allow your body to rest and fully digest nutrients from the day without further burdening your system.

Lay off the caffeine, especially after 2 pm.
Caffeine incites your adrenal glands to produce more adrenaline and cortisol, which keeps you awake.

Avoid alcohol at night.
Drinking alcohol at night means that your body doesn't get enough REM sleep, which doesn't allow it to fully rejuvenate!

Meditate.
This greatly lowers your stress load. More on this later!

Use herbs and teas if needed.
Chamomile, valerian, and kava kava are all mild sedatives. Avoid taking melatonin, however, as it can disrupt your ability to produce your own.

Get off technology - at least one hour before bed (90 minutes is even better).
The artificial blue light from electronics triggers your body to produce more "daytime" hormones, such as cortisol, and interrupts your body's preparation for sleep.

Exercise during the day (not before bedtime).
Exercise can help to encourage the "wake up" hormone, cortisol, in the morning along with encouraging a 75% increase in the reparative "deep sleep" stage at night.

Get more sunlight!
Your circadian clock, or sleep cycle, is heavily impacted by the amount of sunlight you receive during the day. Serotonin production is influenced by the amount of sunlight you receive during the day. Speaking of "getting more sunlight," sleep is essential in regulating (and making) a critical nutrient for your body - Vitamin D!

The point of this book is to focus on emotional eating and not sleep. So I've simply hinted at the power of a good night's rest and some impactful solutions. If you would like to know more strategies for getting the best sleep possible, I highly recommend the *Sleep Smarter* book by Shawn Stevenson. (I am not paid to mention this; it's truly an insightful and helpful read.)

⊙ Vitamin D

So here's something fun - vitamin D isn't a vitamin at all! Vitamins are defined as organic (carbon-containing) chemicals that must be obtained from food or dietary sources because they are not produced by the body. However, vitamin D breaks this rule.

While we do not need a high amount of it (indeed too much can be toxic) like other vitamins and we can obtain it from some foods, it must be transformed by the body to be of any use to us! Indeed, our body makes the best, most bio-available vitamin D from sunshine! Sunlight actually increases dopamine receptors in the body!

By this definition, vitamin D is actually a hormone![20] So, when you say "it's just my hormones," you may very well be right (it just might not be the hormone you expect).

You are likely aware that vitamin D helps with calcium absorption (that's why it's added to milk). But you may not know that it activates genes that regulate the immune system and release neurotransmitters. Researchers have found vitamin D receptors in regions of the brain that are linked to depression.[21] These receptors are now known to play a role in mood, learning, memory, motor control, and perhaps social behavior. Research shows that people with low vitamin D (specifically D3, which is the kind obtained through sunlight) levels are 11 times more prone to be depressed than those with normal levels! [22] Serotonin and oxytocin actually require vitamin D for activation in the brain!

⊙ How Much Do You Need?

The daily recommended dose of vitamin D has been elevated to a range between 800 to 1,200 IU (international unit).[23] Roughly 20 minutes in the sun without sunscreen between the hours of 10am and 3pm will provide most people with 1,000 IU of vitamin D.[24] This amount will vary depending on the darkness of your skin, the season, and the amount of skin exposed to sunlight. So you may need a little less time or a little more time sunbathing. Follow up with sunscreen if you plan to be outdoors for longer than 20 minutes.

If getting enough sunlight is difficult for you, increase your consumption of foods that naturally contain vitamin D: wild-caught mackerel (547 IU for 3 ounces), wild-caught salmon (425 IU for 3 ounces), tuna, cod, oysters, shrimp, beef liver, dairy (100 IU in 8 ounces), oatmeal (150 IU in 1 cup), and eggs (41 IU per egg). Or also consider supplementation by taking vitamin D3 (cholecalciferol) in the recommended dosage.

⊙ Hydration

Are you drinking enough water? Your body - including your brain - is about 75% water! When you are dehydrated, your brain actually shrinks. This has a pretty negative effect on your cognitive functions, such as concentrating, remembering, reaction time, mood, and anxiety.

A body water loss of merely 1-2% can impair cognitive performance and mood!(25) A loss of 5% can cause headaches, nausea, and severe fatigue. Symptoms just get worse as dehydration continues (no one survives more than a 15% loss).

But have no fear - there is an easy fix to this, drink more water! Keeping the body and brain hydrated elevates happiness, memory, alertness, and overall vigor. A properly hydrated brain gives you the power to feel your emotions and make calm decisions on how to handle your response to those feelings.

Unfortunately, our bodies don't have a specific mechanism to tell us that they're thirsty. The same area of the brain that tells us we are hungry (the hypothalamus) is the same area that is triggered when we are dehydrated. So it can be confusing to know if it is water or food that you need. But here are a few questions to help you out:

1. *Did I just eat? If the answer is yes, then you're probably not hungry. Drink water.*
2. *How much water have I had today?*
3. *How much time has passed since I peed?*
4. *Is my urine light yellow or dark (dark means you need more water)?*

How Much Water Do You Need?

Here's an easy way to calculate your fluid intake: divide your current body weight by two and drink that number in ounces. For example: a 160-pound woman needs about 80 ounces of liquids. Notice I said liquids, not water. Drinking plain water is certainly the best way to keep your body hydrated, but water can come from many sources. You can drink tea, juice, coconut water, kombucha... any liquid will give you some level of hydration. Your body receives water from vegetables and fruits, too, but that is much harder to measure in ounces.

Your best bet is to drink water, an occasional tea or juice, and eat plenty of produce!

Masssage

If you ever need an excuse to get a massage, you now have it! Massages help with better emotional balance.

It's true. Massage influences the release of oxytocin, serotonin, and dopamine - three of the "happiness" neurotransmitters in our bodies.

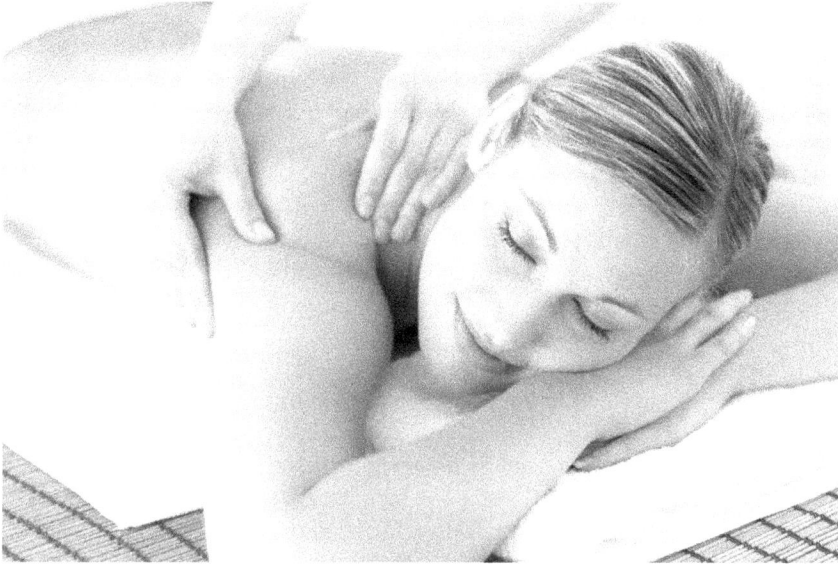

Massage is especially good at activating oxytocin, since it is the "bonding" chemical and is released when we feel a sense of closeness or connectedness to others.

Massage further relaxes you by engaging your parasympathetic nervous system (PSNS). The PSNS is your "relax and recover" nervous system. It is in charge when you are sleeping and engaged when you are fully relaxed. As mentioned already, sleep – high quality sleep – is necessary to maintain balance among emotions. The PSNS increases intestinal and glandular activity (digestion and hormonal balance) in a positive way. If you have a difficult time sleeping or de-stressing, massage may be the answer.

"

If you have a difficult time sleeping or de-stressing, massage may be the answer.

"

Also, when the PSNS is engaged, our sympathetic nervous system (SNS) is disengaged. The sympathetic nervous system is our "fight or flight" response system and is the nervous system that is engaged while we are awake. It is always on the lookout and ready to flee from danger.

The SNS has a powerful ally to cortisol - that pesky stress hormone. By receiving a massage, however, you disengage from the SNS, which automatically lowers cortisol. One study by the National Institutes of Health showed a 31% decrease in cortisol (and a 31% increase in dopamine) in participants following a massage!(26)

But massage has another advantage in supporting an end to emotional eating. Massage connects you to your body in a safe, loving, and non-judgemental space. When you eat emotionally, you are coping and disengaged from yourself. In fact, you may be using food to purposefully not "feel" yourself. By receiving a massage, however, you can reconnect with your body and gain a better understanding of what it needs - what you need - to feel whole and fulfilled without turning to food.

Abdominal massage is particularly powerful in releasing negative emotions, as most of us hold our emotions in our core. Stress/tension goes to the neck and shoulders, anger and worry (for example) go to the belly. But those negative emotions can be flushed away by the flood of dopamine and endorphins released through massage.

Walking

Walking is in the foundations section, because, simply, it's one of the easiest things you can do to help improve your mood and break the emotional eating cycle.

Why bother to move?

Movement is linked to every function in our body. We are in constant movement - lungs expanding, heart pumping, blood flowing, eyes searching. Movement is who we are, yet we sit for most of our days. You sit in a car for a commute, at a desk for work (for 8 to 10 hours sometimes), on the couch when relaxing, in a movie theater, on a park bench. You likely sit more than you realize, and it is impacting your health and your mood.

Movement helps with:

More movement! The muscular system has a "use-it or lose-it" philosophy, losing part of its functionality if a joint or muscle is not used frequently. The less a muscle is used, the harder it is to "get moving" in the future. (It may *even be painful to try.)*

Lymphatic flow. *The lymphatic system is what helps move toxins out of the body and supports a strong immune response. It does not have a pump (like the heart in the cardiovascular system) to function properly and requires physical movement to work effectively.*

Cardiovascular and endocrine systems. *If you want your blood, nutrients, oxygen and hormones to feed your body, regular physical movement aides in the effort.*

Sleep! *Being physically active during the day promotes better quality sleep, less sleep anxiety, and an easier time falling asleep.*

Energy. *Getting "up and at 'em" (as my dad would say) encourages your body to produce its own energy, reducing fatigue, and lethargy.(27)*

Most importantly for this book, movement helps with overall mood elevation and stress reduction. Numerous studies support movement as a means of improving mood and enhancing feelings of well-being. Exercise, especially high intensity exercise, releases endorphins - one of the "feel good" hormones - into the body. Gentler exercise, like walking or yoga, has been associated with a decrease in tension, anxiety, depression, and an improvement in self-esteem.

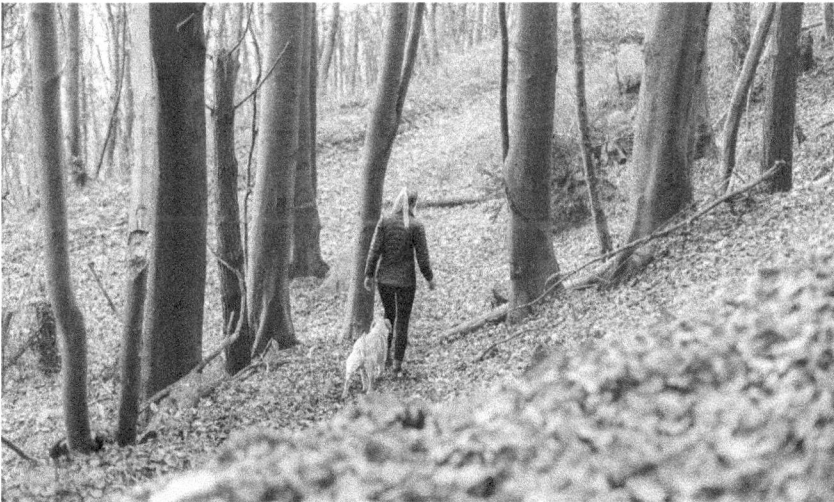

Foundational Solutions

Any type of movement will work, from cleaning the house to dancing to hiking to cross-fit training. I specified walking, because it is easily accessible; it can be done any time of day and just about anywhere without any special equipment.

Take a Nature Walk

If you want to maximize your mood-boosting efforts when you walk, pick a location in nature! A park, a forest, a botanic garden, or even a tree-lined street will benefit your brain. This is because trees (and some other plants) release a chemical called **phytoncides** which have an overall sedative effect on our bodies.(28) Phytoncides appear to greatly reduce stress, ease anxiety, and generally promote relaxation.

There is a beautiful Japanese practice called "shinrin-yoku," which means "taking in the forest atmosphere" or "forest bathing." I love that image! Some of the benefits of forest bathing include:

* *Reduced blood pressure and stress,(29)*
* *Improved mood,*
* *Increased ability to focus,*
* *Boosted immune system functioning,*
* *Increased energy levels, and*
* *Improved sleep.*

How long do you need to walk?

A nice long walk will do wonders, but if you are pressed for time, 30 minutes of movement a day is all you need for overall well-being (especially if you are used to sitting more than moving). Even better yet, you only need to move for 12 minutes to see improvement in joy, vigor, self-confidence, and focus!

Mindful Eating

So this piece is super important, and I could write a whole book just on this topic (indeed many have). Here is why it is so important: *when you are eating emotionally, you are eating mindlessly.*

Mindful simply means "aware" or "paying attention to." Therefore, mindful eating means that you are eating with awareness. You are focused on the experience of eating with all of your senses and attention.

In contrast, emotional eating is often about filling emptiness or uncertainty, taking away the pain and discomfort, or getting away from the emotion because "who has time to deal with it anyway."

It is mindless.

It is grabbing the bag of potato chips, sitting in front of the TV, eating, and then suddenly realizing the bag is empty when you try to grab another handful. It's eating a pint of ice cream at night as you flip through social media. It's an escape.

By practicing mindful eating, you can put an end to eating patterns that do not support your overall well-being. Notice I said "practicing." Mindful eating is an easy process but can be difficult to adopt because it requires you to do two key things: (1) slow down and savor and (2) tune in to your feelings.

The first step - slowing down - is hard enough. We live in a "go, go, go!" society, which is true whether you work full time or are a stay-at-home parent. The to-dos are ever present, and time is fleeting. **But I encourage**

you to pause. Just stop for a brief moment and take a deep breath. Ask yourself: "Why am I about to eat this food?" Is it hunger or something else? Allow the emotion or thought to surface. Listen to what your body has to say.

If it's hunger, then eat mindfully. If it's an emotional need, then eat mindfully. Or don't eat... but be mindful of that choice! **Be aware of the why** behind your actions and decisions.

Now when you are ready to eat, really **savor** your food. Whatever the food is! One wonderful thing in mindful eating is the elimination of judgement about our food items. There are no "bad" or "good" foods in mindful eating. There are "sometimes" and "always" foods.*(30)* Cheetos are a **sometimes** foods, while a piece of real, whole cheddar is an **always** food. French fries are a **sometimes** food, while a baked sweet potato is an **always** food.

By adopting the practice of sometimes and always foods, you automatically eliminate the possibility of guilt or shame (remember the guilt and shame cycle discussed earlier) from your diet. You are not a bad person because you ate a "bad" food. You are a human being who decided to eat a sometimes food. In that **one** moment. The next moment, you can be a human being who decides to eat an always food. Don't let the "good/bad" foods create judgement that leads to more emotional eating!

But let's get back to the idea of **Savoring**.

One issue with emotional eating is that, since it is mindless in nature, you are not really aware of your food. It's just a bandaid used to get through something else. By savoring your food, you give your body and mind time to register the food - time to be aware.

Savoring involves eating with all your senses - touch, smell, taste, sight, and yes, even hearing.

After all, we eat for reasons that aren't always emotional. We eat because:

* *Something sounds good (fajitas)*
* *Something smells good (popcorn)*
* *Something looks good (chocolate lava cake)*
* *Some "thing" told me I should (a billboard, a TV commercial, an app)*

Our senses play a huge role in moderating our eating activities and decisions. Take the time to engage those senses when eating. **Follow these steps to savor:**

Take one bite at a time. *Pick up one piece or one small bite of your food.*

1. **Look at it carefully.** *Look at the texture, the color, the shape. Look at it as if you have never seen this food before (which if you think about it, you haven't, or at least not this exact one).*
2. **Bring it to your nose, and smell it.** *Studies show that smell has a dominant role in flavor (it is said that 80% of taste comes from smell, but that is now shown to be difficult to actually quantify).(31) And our ability to distinguish flavors (bitterness vs. sweetness for example) begins with smell!(32)*
3. **Feel it.** *Place the food in your mouth but do not chew yet. Feel its texture with your tongue.*
4. **Begin chewing.** *Slowly chew the food. Embrace your inner sloth! Your saliva has different digestive enzymes than your stomach. Chewing not only allows your brain the time to register all the distinct flavors that may be present, it allows your body to start digesting the food and absorbing key nutrients, making your stomach's job much easier. Most people chew 3 to 5 times, which really stresses your gut. Try for 15, 20, or even 30 chews per bite! It's harder than it sounds but offers great benefit to your body.*
5. **Taste.** *While chewing, really pay attention to taste. Is it bitter or sweet, salty or bland? Does the taste change as you eat? Do you even like the taste of this food? That may seem like a silly question, but on several occasions, I've had clients say, "Wow, I don't even like that food. I've always eaten it because my mom served it, but I really don't like the flavor!"*
6. **Swallow.** *Be aware of the sensation of swallowing. Be aware that your body has just consumed a small amount of energy and nutrients. Were those nutrients beneficial to your body? Did you get enough energy or do you need more?*
7. **Repeat.** *Continue eating mindfully until you feel satiated (fully satisfied). Pay attention to your level of hunger and fullness as you eat and stop eating when you are pleasantly full (not unbuttoning your pants like it's Thanksgiving) and no longer hungry.*
8. **Check in.** *Is your body happy and content? Is your mind eased from the emotional trigger?*

Which brings us to the second step, **Tuning In.**

Mindful eating is slow and intentional, giving you the space to tune into your feelings, giving space for emotions to take form and become tangible.

Being present with your emotions may feel scary at first. You may feel incapable of dealing with your feelings head on or of facing hard realities. You feel powerless over your emotions, so you eat... You have power over that, right? But then you start to feel that you are powerless over food and begin to eat because "there's nothing you can do"... and it does make you feel better.

But the truth is, when you don't try to suppress, ignore, or hide from your emotions they lose their power over you. Even the most painful feelings ease and relent when you allow them to just be; when you can accept them as a part of you. Think, "Oh, I have lungs, I have a stomach, I have two eyes and ten fingers and a bunch of emotions too."

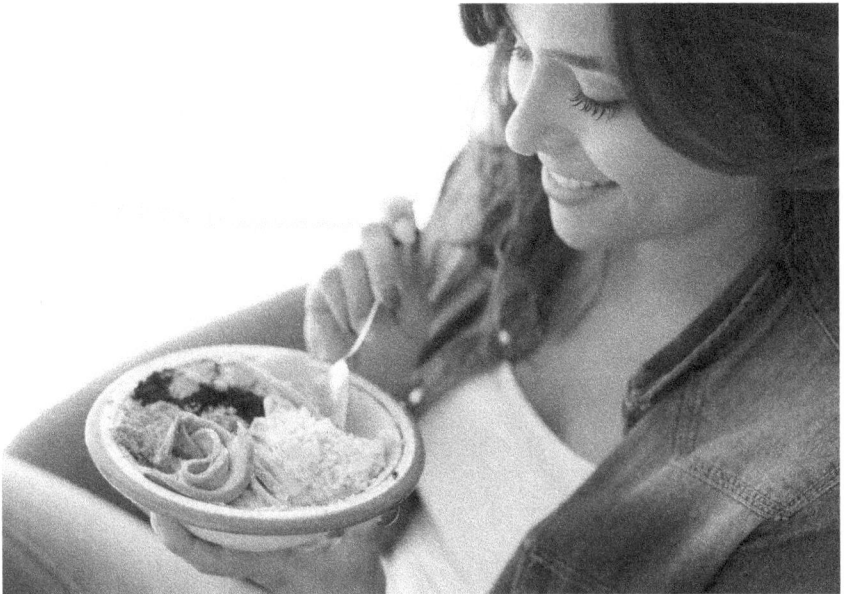

To tune in, pay attention as you eat, allowing yourself to be present with whatever emotion arises. With gentle curiosity, examine that emotion. Where does it come from? Why is it there? What is it teaching you? Perhaps your day, or just that specific moment, called up something from your past where food helped you to feel better.

Think like a scientist conducting an experiment. There are variables - A causes B. The scientist will change the variables and observe the results... all with a detached inquisitiveness. You can do this too, simply by observing your emotions and considering the "variables." Then, what happens if you change a variable?

You may realize that you are eating because you are lonely after work. So change the variable - meet friends for a walk after work or join a social group. How does that change your emotional eating?

You may realize that you are eating because you are deeply frustrated with your job. Change the variable; can you find a new job? Will that ease the desire to eat?

You are completely **in control** of the variables and your actions or reactions. But you can only make healthy and balanced choices once you have an **awareness** of yourself. As Sir Francis Bacon once said, "Knowledge is power." Indeed it is - power over your food cravings. Power to change your habits. Power to love yourself!

"

You are completely in control of the variables and your actions or reactions. But you can only make healthy and balanced choices once you have an awareness of yourself.

"

Awareness comes through eating mindfully... just one bite at a time. And one breath at a time...

Aromatherapy

Speaking of breathing, you may want to consider diffusing some essential oils into the air. Our sense of smell is the only sense directly tied to the limbic area of the brain, which is also known as our emotional and memory control center. (Other senses must first be routed through the thalamus in the brain.) This means that smell is powerful in influencing your emotions. It is also why certain smells can bring a memory rushing back to the surface.

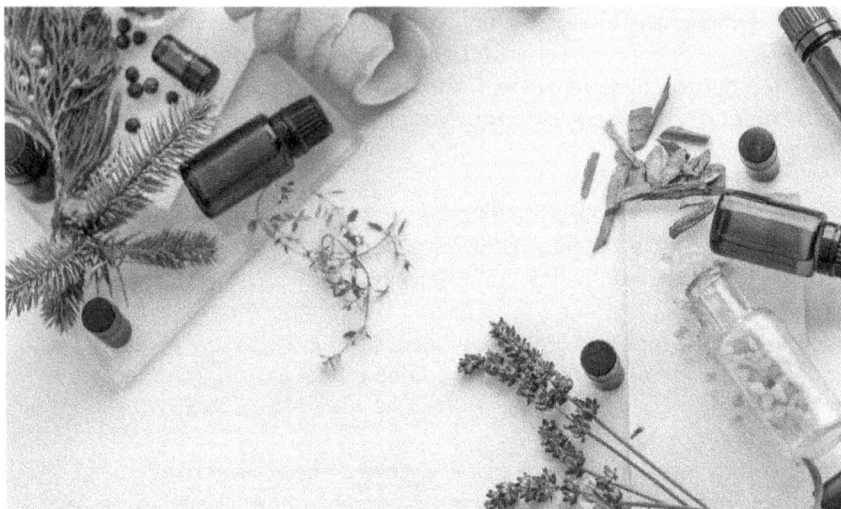

I know whenever I smell freshly baked bread, I am reminded of my mom's holiday rolls, and when I smell pipe tobacco, I am transported to my great-grandfather's living room.

Smell can be powerful in affecting what and how much we eat as well. One study by J. A. Reed et al. shows that peppermint scent can be effective in decreasing appetite and hunger cravings and in consuming fewer calories.*(33)* Other studies have shown a decrease in hunger and cravings from smelling green apple, banana, vanilla, or even extra virgin olive oil!

All scents will have an influence on your mind and body. Explore this experience by:

- *Diffusing essential oils.*
- *Lighting an aromatherapy candle made from 100% soy, beeswax, coconut wax, hemp oil, or some other combination that doesn't contain any paraffin.*
- *Cooking with herbs and spices.*
- *Visiting a botanic garden.*
- *Taking a hike through a pine forest.*

In the Food for Feelings section of this book, I have listed beneficial essential oils for each emotion. Now that you know why breathing is so important to your emotions, let's take a look at *how* to breathe.

⊙ Connect with Breathing: Everyday and Meditate

While breathing seems like an obvious choice to be in the foundations section of this book, you may be wondering why I have to bring it up? Don't we all naturally breathe? Yes, hopefully! But there are different ways of breathing that can make a big impact on your ability to ease your emotions and remain more balanced.

Let's address two types of breathing: (1) diaphragmatic and (2) meditative.

Diaphragmatic breathing is breathing from your diaphragm (pretty simple, I know). But most people tend to breathe from their chest, drawing air into the lungs by opening the rib cage. This actually limits the capacity of the lungs and causes the neck and shoulder muscles to constrict in an effort to "lift" and help to open the ribcage. Ouch! This is shallow breathing.

Shallow breathing further engages the sympathetic nervous system which keeps you in a stressed state. But when you breathe deeply, by drawing air in and "down" by way of the diaphragm, then you help the body to engage that parasympathetic nervous system and immediately begin to relax!

Try it now - allow your belly to expand with three deep breaths and feel your neck and shoulders release, your body tension lessen and a sense of calm fill your body and mind. Make breathing this way as your new norm!

Meditative breathing is much more involved. It requires focus and practice. But it, too, is accessible to everyone, and I can say from firsthand experience that it's a life changer.

I'll admit that I was never one to meditate until fairly recently. I grew up believing meditation to be pretty "woo-woo" and something to avoid if I wanted to "fit in." Then I thought "I don't have time" or "It's too hard" or "I'll never get my mind to be empty." Boy, was I wrong! Meditation has become a necessity in my life, just like...well, *breathing*. And there is always time - just 10 minutes a day can have tremendous results. It's not hard once you've practiced a bit. And it's not about having an empty mind. It's about being present with your mind, but not following it down the rabbit hole!

Do you recall that inner critic I mentioned earlier? The one that keeps telling you "you're not worthy?" Meditation helps to silence that negative voice. Oh, the voice will still be there, but you can push it aside and allow the other "voice" - the inner guide - to have a platform to speak. The inner guide tells you, "You are worth so very much, and you are capable and beautiful!" It's a lovely voice to hear.

Science Supports Meditation

Due to research by neuroscientists and advancements in technology, scientists and the broader medical community now embrace meditation (and mindfulness) as a concrete way to increase health and overall wellbeing.

Studies have shown that meditation actually **changes** your brain! During meditation, the brain increases in grey matter, which is involved in muscle control, sensory perception, memory, emotions, decision-making, and self-control. Additionally, meditation increases the brain's volume in the regions associated with creating habits and emotional stability.(34) Overall, the brain changes, giving you better self-control, better emotional regulation, more positive feelings, and stronger decision-making capabilities.

Outside of structural changes, meditation has a positive influence on all the systems in the body. You have:

- Increased immunity,(35)
- Decreased inflammation and pain,
- Increased focus and alertness,
- Improved digestion,
- Reduced anxiety and stress,(36)
- Increased feelings of life satisfaction,
- Increased positive emotions, and
- More feelings of social connectedness and life purpose.

There are plenty more benefits to list, but do you really need more?

Meditation and Emotional Eating

Your inner guide - the voice of wisdom - can also be thought of as your "inner mind." Your outer mind is super chatty. It's planning, analyzing, judging, or just plain filling up the silence. But your inner mind is calm, patient, and speaks only when given the space, or the opening, to speak.

Mindfulness meditation allows the inner mind to take control **instead of your habitual patterns**. The purpose of meditation is to train your capacity to observe the experience of both the body and the mind, slowly bringing more conscious control over your thoughts, feelings, and automatic reactions.

Meditation provides a few minutes of quiet in order to just observe rather than react, to drop into the deeper, wiser parts of our minds which may be hard to access when we are stressed, irritated, or upset.

Meditation allows emotions to come forward. It allows you a space to just sit with them and be with your feelings to mindfully experience them more clearly. It also makes room for more positive thoughts and feelings to emerge, where once they may have been overshadowed by the negative ones.

When you are in more control of yourself, you can more easily "ride out" negative emotions. This is called "**surfing the urge**." It means that when an emotion arises, rather than immediately grabbing your favorite food, you can surf that feeling for a moment and see if it naturally passes away. You can ride that emotion to its conclusion, which may not involve a need for food at all!

Or think of it this way: Imagine a lovely beach with waves rolling in. The wave starts at the surface, gathers volume, rises high into the air, and then topples over and disappears. Our emotions are much like that wave - starting to surface, gaining intensity, bubbling up, and then over to disappear. If you can surf that wave, well you can master your emotions and surf through life.

> **When you are in more control of yourself, you can more easily "ride out" negative emotions.
> This is called "surfing the urge."**

How to Meditate

Meditation takes practice. Thankfully though, there is no right or wrong way to meditate. (There are ways that are more effective than others, but you have choices and can find what works for you.) The important thing is to meditate daily. Make this a habit so you can use it when needed. The more you practice, the easier it is for you to connect to your inner mind and inner calm.

Think of an activity or sport that you wanted to be really good at. How did you get good? It's doubtful that you wished on a shooting star and the next morning you were a star soccer player. (If that worked, though, major high five!) More likely, you woke up every day, put on your soccer shoes and practiced drills, up and down the field.

Consider meditation as another sport or hobby. It may be hard to start at first, but once you get over the stumbles and the hurdles, once you daily set time aside to focus, you will get better and better. You will gain the effects of greater awareness, relaxation, and control in your life, especially where you really need it - throughout the day and when eating.

To begin, find a place that is quiet and comfortable. Sit in a relaxed position. (Sitting is better than lying down, as you may fall asleep.) Gently close your eyes and focus on your breathing. **Just your breath.** Other thoughts (that outer chatter) will pop into your mind. Simply acknowledge it as "just a thought" and return to your breathing. Try to do this for 10 minutes to begin with, eventually working your way up to 20 or more minutes per day.

You don't have to do this alone - there are a ton of recorded (guided) meditations online. Just search for "Mindfulness Meditation," which will be a terrific place to start if you are just beginning. Also, if you are looking for a guided meditation that specifically helps with eating, visit The Center for Mindful Eating's website for free resources.

Here is a simple technique that you can use anytime, anywhere to refocus and center. I call it the **"Mindful Minute."**

Find a comfortable place to sit (or stand if necessary) and gently close your eyes.

Connect with your diaphragm for long deep breaths:

Breathe in for a slow count of 4.

Breathe out to a slow count of 6.

Repeat this 6 times then gently open your eyes.

You've just completed one minute of mindfulness!

Now don't you feel more positive? Let's keep that going!

Positive Mindset

Emotional eating tends to default to, and stem from, negative thoughts. There are several versions of a quote that I love: "What you focus on expands." Good or bad, it grows.

I remember when I took a motorcycle driver's ed class. The instructor was teaching us about safety and how to avoid potholes, rocks, squirrels, etc. One thing in particular that stuck with me was when he said: "If you see a boulder in the road, you'll want to get around it, so don't look at it! Look at where you **want** to go and you'll go there. Keep your eyes to the side of the boulder, look to the path around the rock and you will go there. Look at the boulder, and you'll go there too!" At first I thought he was crazy, but now I get it. If I focused on the boulder, than it just expanded in my mind, getting bigger and impossible to avoid. What you focus on expands.

It is a powerful statement in life. If you focus on the negative thoughts, then they will get bigger and feel heavier, becoming all consuming. If you continually tell yourself that you are bad for eating out of control, then you will keep finding ways to reinforce that belief. If you are always focused on food, then food will always be front and center in your life.

Good news though - this works in reverse too! What if that focus was positive? If you focused on positive thoughts, then positivity would grow. If you focused on how amazing and beautiful you are, then, well you couldn't help yourself, you'd be forced to become more amazing and beautiful!

There's a super simple way to make a positive mindset part of your life, and that's to begin a **Gratitude Practice**.

Be Grateful

Gratitude is a way of affirming the good things in your life. Gratitude practice is linked to better mental health and life satisfaction(37) as grateful people experience more joy, love and enthusiasm! Regularly expressing gratitude reduces depression, anxiety, and blood pressure. Grateful people cope better with stress, recover faster from illness, have better immune function, and enjoy more overall physical health! They are also protected from envy, greed, bitterness, and sadness. All this from giving thanks!

Showing gratitude further releases our happiness chemicals: dopamine as a reward for finding something good, serotonin for motivation to do it again, and oxytocin for the social connection when gratitude is expressed towards or for others.(38)

Those feel good chemicals reduce unpleasant feelings. Negative emotional states make it difficult to regulate your eating. The more you practice gratitude, or being thankful, the more your mind stays in a positive mindset, making it easier for you to adopt healthy habits like making better eating choices and not self-soothing with food. Anger, guilt, sadness - all those negative emotions cannot thrive in a positive environment. Your negative emotions take a backseat to the positive ones.

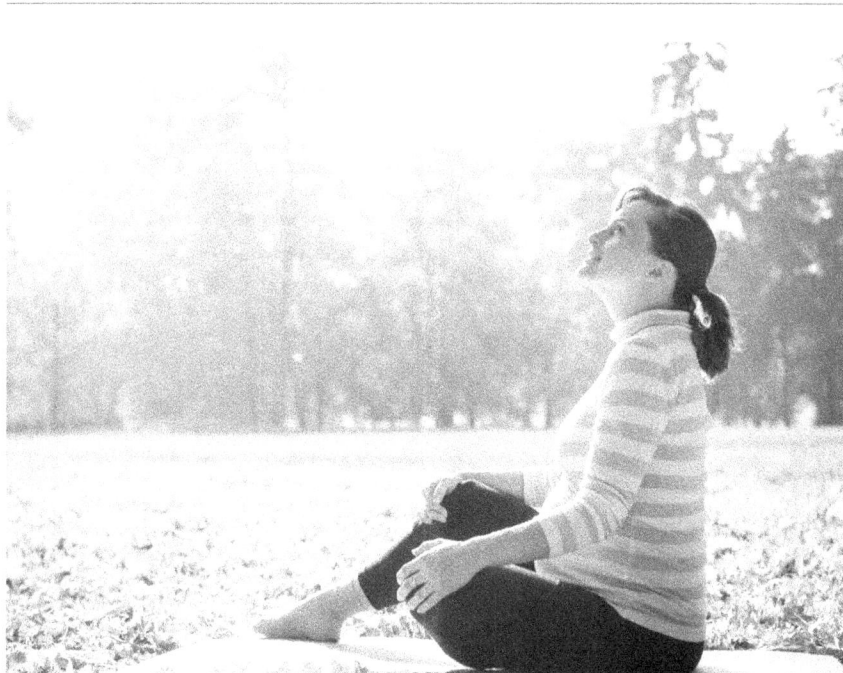

This doesn't happen immediately however. Our brains are hardwired by habit. We talked about those learned behaviors and that eating cookies or nachos when you are sad was likely established while you were a child or teenager. In neuroscience, Hebb's law states that "nerves that fire together, wire together." The more you can activate the "gratitude circuits" in the brain, the stronger those neural pathways will become! So to reap the benefits of gratitude, you have to practice giving thanks every day!

You know how easy it can be to focus on the bad stuff: "my belly's too big, my boss is mean, I'm not a good mom." That's because those neural networks have been travelled many times and are easily activated. It's comfortable for your brain to travel the same path.

But our brain likes a good challenge, too, so it has "neuroplasticity," or an ability to adapt and change. By understanding Hebb's law, we know that if we continually fire the grateful neurons, then those will become hardwired and will be the new preferred path for our thoughts!

Ways to Be Grateful

A gratitude practice can be anything you like. It simply needs to engage your brain in searching for "moments of thanks" and allow you to express that gratitude. Here are some suggestions:

1. **Keep a gratitude journal.** *Each evening before bed, write down three things that you are grateful for. They can be as simple as coffee or as complex as forgiving an old friend. Don't overthink it! The act of seeking releases the feel good chemicals.*

2. **Smile.** *Smile to others as you meet them on the street. Smile at your barista or grocery clerk. Others will feel your kindness and joy, and they too will smile. Then, before you know it, gratitude spreads like wildfire!*

3. **Show random acts of kindness.** *Doing nice things or giving gifts to others really ups the game in gratitude. You feel great showing kindness to others; they feel great receiving kindness. Doing it for no particular reason releases more dopamine than if you "had" to do something (buy a Christmas gift for example).*

4. **Write a letter.** *Find someone to whom you'd like to express thanks and send them a letter. It's a powerful way to rewire your brain for gratitude.*

Final thought on gratitude: **Fine tune your perspective**. We cannot always control what happens to us in life, but we can control our reactions. If you are happy or sad, it's all in the way you perceive the moment. Even a difficult moment or situation can be a valuable learning experience. You may not realize it in the moment but be open to realizing it in the future.

For example losing a job may feel depressing and terrifying. But if you can shift your perspective a bit from, "This is terrible! My life is ruined!" to "Well, this sucks, but what can I learn from this so I can find a better job?", you can stay hardwired to that positive neural pathway even in difficult times. Perspective can give you strength to make better decisions or keep you locked in place.

Shifting perspective can change your desire to eat when those negative emotions arise. Remember, what you focus on expands - so where do you want your focus to be?! For now, though, let's focus on finding the best food to help your feelings.

Foods for Feelings

Let's Get Specific

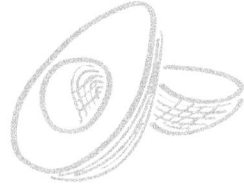

How to Use This Section

The following chapters are broken into emotions that we regularly feel which may also prompt us to eat. I've found that most emotional eating occurs between meals, during the times when we are looking to "fill the void." Food can be very filling! So the recipes here focus on snack-type or quick foods - foods that you can quickly grab, make, or take on the go.

I've also tried to make these recipes super simple, using ingredients that you can find, buy, and "slap together." For example, in the chicken salad recipe there is mayonnaise. Yes, it's likely healthier to make your own, but homemade mayonnaise is not usually a priority for most of us (certainly isn't one of mine). So select the best quality ingredients that you can without losing your mind.

Helpful foods are also listed, so you know which ones can better support your emotions during meal times as well. These lists are not exhaustive but contain foods that are commonly eaten.

Also keep in mind a basic rule of "5." **You should strive for five servings of fruits and vegetables everyday.** Try to eat as much produce as possible to improve your emotional balance (and overall health). Here's a major reason why:

*   Dopamine is a primary neurotransmitter behind feeling good. Foods in the following chapters contain the amino acids tyrosine and phenylalanine, which convert into dopamine. Vitamins C, B-6, and

folic acid, as well as the minerals zinc, copper, magnesium, iron, and manganese must be present for this conversion. Likewise, the B vitamins are also essential for the optimal use of dopamine in the body.*(39)*

- Dopamine converts into norepinephrine (which is opposite of adrenaline) and additional vitamin C is needed to make that happen.*(40)*

If you are eating your five servings of a variety of produce, you should easily be able to meet the demand for vitamins and minerals to support your feel good chemicals.

One word (ok several) on supplements. Supplements should be just that - supplemental to your diet. You can take a multivitamin to receive your vitamins and minerals, but you will be missing out on all the wonderful antioxidants, fiber, phytonutrients, and trace minerals that your body needs as well. If you plan to use a supplement, select a high quality, whole-food sourced product. The higher cost is usually well worth it as supplements can range from little more than a sugar pill to a bio-available nutrient. The FDA does not oversee quality control on supplements, so do your research!

Also in this section, you'll find suggestions for "non-food" activities and exercises, along with questions for self-reflection.

Special thanks is given to **yoga instructor, Mindy Arbuckle and personal trainer, Daniel Hall** for providing their expertise in yoga and exercise. They took time to identify specific yoga poses and exercises that can help with each emotion and the eating urges they lead to. Use these movements to help "surf the urge" when a food craving hits. Keep in mind that you will gain the most benefit from practicing these movements regularly so that when you need them for specific purposes, they will be familiar and aid you more thoroughly.

Remember, these are foods and steps that can help, but you only need to **take one step at a time.** Perhaps you can do all the suggestions and have an amazing day (or week)! Or perhaps you can only manage to choose roasted almonds over an Almond Joy. Listen to your body and promise to treat yourself gently but also make the promise to **do** - **do** make a small change, **do** take a next step, **do** try something different, **do** better than the day before. You are on your way to freedom from emotional eating! Choose your emotion and begin your journey.

⊙ Boredom

Whenever I ask, "What emotions are a trigger for you?", 90% of the time "Boredom" is the response. As an emotion, this one is a bit difficult to pinpoint. It's a mixture of a lack of satisfaction and a low level of desire to do anything. We even struggle with how to define it as a feeling, usually just settling on, "I'm just bored." But it's a powerful feeling. **It is one that makes us grab whatever is available and just start eating.** We stop eating when we are no longer bored but is that because we figured out a better way to fill our time or is it because of a chemical shift in the brain? Perhaps, it's both.

Scientists have noticed that boredom-prone people naturally have lower levels of dopamine.(41) This means that, if you are often bored, you need more stimulus to excite your brain.

Interestingly, people who have damage to their brain's frontal cortex tend to be more prone to boredom. This suggests that the frontal cortex plays a major role in feelings of boredom. This same area of the brain also controls our perception of time and could be linked to the sensation of time passing more slowly.

Eating passes the time, certainly. Choosing foods that help to increase dopamine levels could resolve your boredom more quickly.

Chemical in charge: dopamine (too little)

Foods that can help

With boredom, protein is your friend. These foods are rich in tyrosine, which boosts dopamine levels. Choose:

- Meat: Grass-fed beef, pasture-raised chicken or turkey, pasture-raised eggs, Bison, lean pork
- Wild-caught fish, especially salmon (high in Omega-3) or tuna
- Dairy (animal)
- Yogurt
- Nuts and seeds, especially pumpkin seeds, sesame seeds, and peanuts
- Fruit, specifically bananas, apples, cranberries, strawberries, apricots, and peaches
- Avocados
- Beans, especially lima beans
- Grains, specifically wild rice and oats
- Olives
- Beets
- Artichokes
- Dark chocolate

Activities that can help

- Calling a friend (be social)
- Having a "go-to" list of things to get done - start to check those off!
- Dancing! Turn on your favorite song and shake your booty!

Essential Oils

- Peppermint
- Orange (citrus blends)

Exercises/movement that can help

- Try a new class (Zumba, pilates, barre, belly dancing... What excites you?)
- Speed skating
- Stair step-ups
- Just get moving - do 15 squats, lunge across your living room, or do 25 jumping jacks. Get oxygen flowing and let the happiness chemicals release!

Helpful Yoga poses

- Cat Cow
- Happy Baby
- Robins Breath
- Side Plank
- Side Crow
- Extended Side Angle

Extended Side Angle

Healthy snack recipes

With boredom, you are looking for something to do, so this is a great time to select snacks which need assembling, prep work or creativity.

- Chicken Salad with Crackers
- Quinoa with Beets, Goat Cheese, and Apples
- Deli Meat Wraps
- Homemade Trail Mix

Reflect and Journal

- Are you truly bored or simply trying to avoid a situation or something/someone?
- Are there activities that you enjoy doing which could fill your time (or, are there other ways to replace your boredom)? Maybe you have a hobby or talent which has taken a backseat and could be become a part of your life once again?
- Is there an area in your life in which you are lacking satisfaction? Are there ways to increase your satisfaction levels in that area?

Recipes

Deli Meat Wrap

Ingredients
- 2 slices of deli meat of your choice (select nitrate/nitrite-free meats)
- Sliced vegetables of your choice
- Sliced cheese of your choice (optional)

Instructions
Place vegetables and cheese on the far edge of the deli meat, and roll until it forms a wrap. Here are some of my favorites:

- Ham, cheddar, pickles, drizzle of mustard
- Turkey, hummus, bell peppers
- Turkey, spinach, avocado
- Roast beef, swiss, arugula, drizzle of mustard

Chicken Salad with Crackers

Ingredients
- 1 can (8 to 12 oz) chicken breast in water, drained (I really enjoy Harvest Creek brand of organic chicken. You can also use leftover rotisserie or grilled chicken)
- Handful (maybe 12) of red or green grapes, sliced in half
- 2 scallions, thinly sliced
- 1 celery stalk, thinly sliced
- 1/2 cup of mixed baby greens or baby spinach
- 1/4 cup slivered almonds
- 1 tbsp pumpkin seeds
- 1/4 to 1/3 cup mayonnaise
- Salt and pepper to taste
- Dash of dried dill or cayenne (optional)
- ~10 whole grain, rice, or nut crackers

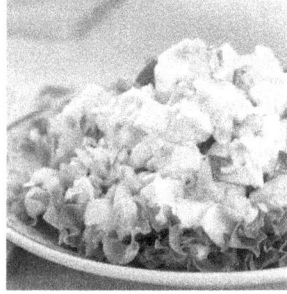

Instructions
Combine all ingredients (accept for the crackers) in a bowl. Adjust ingredients to taste (maybe you need more grapes or seeds for example). Eat with your favorite cracker (avoid saltines or over processed crackers). I enjoy eating Crunchmaster brand multi-grain, gluten-free crackers or Nut-Thins brand crackers. Yes - you can eat this with bread, but the crackers allow you to "dip" into the chicken salad for a quick snack, rather than building a full sandwich. Keep leftovers in an airtight container in the fridge.

Quinoa with Beets, Goat Cheese, and Apples

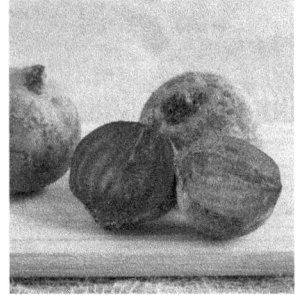

Ingredients
- 1 cup quinoa
- 4 small beets, diced
- 1/4 to 1/3 cup of toasted walnuts, crushed
- 1/2 green apple, diced
- Herbed goat cheese, crumbled
- Dressing: 2 oz Golden balsamic vinegar
- 1 oz Maple syrup

Instructions
1. Follow cooking instructions for the quinoa. Set aside to let cool.
2. For the beets, you can either open a jar of quality pickled beets (fastest method) or purchase raw beets and roast them following the instructions below.
3. In a bowl, mix together the diced apple and walnuts. In a separate dish blend the vinegar and maple syrup. *These are "to taste": you can use more or less depending on your liking.
4. Once the beets and quinoa are cooled, add them to the bowl with the apples and walnuts. Add goat cheese, as much as you like (I use about half of a 5 oz log). Pour dressing over the mixture and stir. If you cannot find herbed goat cheese, use plain goat cheese and add dried basil, rosemary, and thyme (or your favorite herbs).

Roasting beets:
1. Preheat oven to 400 degrees.
2. If the beets still have their leafy tops, cut off the tops close to the tops of the beet. Scrub the beets thoroughly, then wrap them loosely in aluminum foil. No need to dry the beets before wrapping. Small beets can be wrapped together, but it's easiest to roast large beets individually.
3. Place the wrapped beets on a rimmed baking sheet to catch drips in case the juices leak. Roast for 50 to 60 minutes. Check the beets every 20 minutes or so. If they are starting to look dry or are scorching on the bottoms, dribble a tablespoon of water over the beets before re-wrapping. Beets are done when a fork or skewer slides easily to the center of the beet. Small beets will cook more quickly than large beets.

Homemade Trail Mix

If you are bored, but still in a hurry, you can certainly buy pre-made trail mixes. There are a myriad of combinations that are readily available. However, if you have the time, making your own trail mix is easy and can help to ease that feeling of boredom quickly.

Ingredients
- 1 cup of your favorite nuts, toasted or roasted
- 1/2 cup of your favorite dried fruit
- 1/2 cup seeds
- 1/2 cup dark chocolate

Adjust quantity to your liking; plan ahead and prepare larger batches. Save money by purchasing raw nuts in bulk.

Instructions to Roasting Nuts
1. Soak the nuts in water for 2 hours, then rinse and dry thoroughly
2. Preheat oven to 350 degrees
3. Place whole nuts in a single layer on a baking sheet
4. Bake 5 to 10 minutes or until they are golden brown
5. Remove and let cool

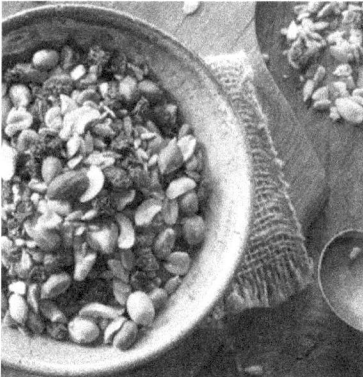

Boredom Buster Trail Mix
Almonds, cashews, banana chips, apple bits, pumpkin seeds, dark chocolate

⊙ Depression

Depression - this is a heavy word that carries the burden of many emotions. The problem is that the emotions are "depressed," and often the concern is that you can't **feel** any emotions. You are simply down, or in a depressed state, and nothing excites you.

Let's make an important distinction here - there is a difference between being sad and being depressed. Sadness happens all the time and is a perfectly normal emotion to a trigger that is hurtful, difficult, or challenging. Sometimes sadness just needs a good cry to feel better.

Depression, on the other hand, is much more complicated and usually does not require a trigger to cause the depressed state. It shades every aspect of your life and saps your motivation and energy.(42) At its best, it is a state of mind that is lacking in proper nutrition and exercise for the brain to function properly. At its worst, it is a mental illness that affects all areas of your life in pervasive and chronic ways.

I include depression in this book, because it's common for people to say, "I'm not sure what's wrong. I'm just depressed." After looking into their diets, I can see that they are malnourished and lacking any support in their systems to be happy. But, if you feel that your depression is chronic - a daily occurrence that doesn't change with any support - please seek medical attention. Sometimes diet alone cannot overcome depression!

The solutions offered below are intended to help with mild to moderate depressed states, not chronic depression.

Chemical in charge: norepinephrine (low), serotonin (low), dopamine (low), cortisol (high)

Foods that can help

- Turmeric* (1,500 mg) - quality and quantity matters here. In studies, curcumin (the active ingredient in tumeric) worked as powerfully as Prozac. However, you must take a bioavailable form or take tumeric with pepper (peperine). Otherwise, your body only absorbs about 2% of the curcumin!
- Protein - all (beans, nuts, dairy)
- Soy (which is a phytoestrogen, so limit consumption)
- Eggs
- Cheese
- Quinoa
- Wheat germ
- Whole grains
- Leafy greens
- Red/orange/yellow bell peppers
- Papaya
- Bananas
- Watermelon
- Oranges
- Cantaloupe
- Broccoli
- Red cabbage
- Nuts
- Pumpkin and squash seeds
- Oats
- Arctic root (Rhodiola rosea) (adaptogenic herb)*
- Ginseng or euthero (adaptogenic herb)*
- Dark Chocolate

These can affect medications, so consult with your doctor before implementing them into any changes in your diet.

Activities that can help

- Playing with temperature - a cold plunge or shower or sitting in a sauna significantly raises norepinephrine levels
- Getting a pet for a companion (but only if its care excites you and doesn't burden you)
- Gardening
- Volunteering to do something you love
- Reading a book
- Listening to music or a fun podcast

Essential Oils

- Lavender
- Ylang Ylang

Exercises/movement that can help

- Bicycle riding
- Yoga or Tai Chi
- Jogging/running
- Bear Crawl
- Superman

Superman

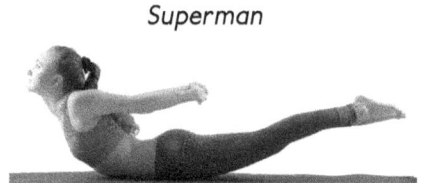

Helpful Yoga poses

- Camel
- Cobra
- Supported Fish
- Warrior 1
- Handstand
- Tree

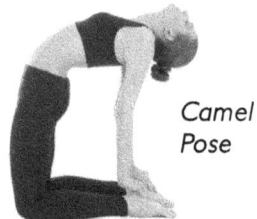

Camel Pose

Healthy snack recipes

- Golden Milk
- Blissful Nut Butter Toast
- Hummus with Bell Peppers
- Happiness in a Bowl: Fruit Salad and Cheese

Reflect and Journal

- Is a situation causing your depression? Can you change that situation?
- Is a person affecting your depression? Is this a person you need to keep in your life? Can you change the relationship in a positive way?
- Is your schedule overloaded? What can you delegate or remove from your responsibilities? With whom can you share the load?

Recipes

Blissful Nut Butter Toast

Ingredients
- 3 tbsp almond butter (or your favorite nut butter)
- 1 tsp raw, unfiltered honey
- 1 tsp chia seeds
- 1/2 tsp ground flax seeds
- 1 tbsp raw cocoa nibs
- ~1 tbsp coconut oil
- 1/2 banana
- 1 slice of sourdough bread (or whole grain bread)

Instructions
Blend the first five ingredients above together in a small bowl and set aside. Toast the bread in a toaster. While still warm, spread the coconut oil over the toast (start with a knifeful and add more if needed). Spread a thin layer of the nut butter mixture over the toast. Top with sliced banana (add as much banana as you like). The remaining nut butter will keep well in the fridge. Enjoy!

Golden Milk

(recipe courtesy of Dr. Weil and available at drweil.com along with an instructional video)

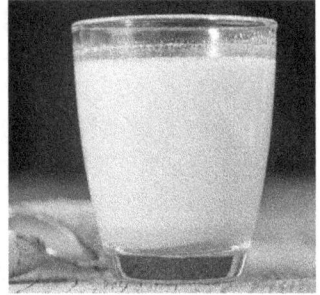

Ingredients
- 2 cups light, unsweetened coconut milk
- 1/2 tablespoon peeled, grated fresh ginger
- 1 tablespoon peeled, grated fresh turmeric
- 3-4 black peppercorns

Instructions
1. Heat 2 cups light, unsweetened coconut milk (or your favorite milk/milk substitue)
2. Add ½ tablespoon peeled, grated fresh ginger
3. Add 1 tablespoon peeled, grated fresh turmeric
4. Add 3-4 black peppercorns
5. Heat all ingredients in a saucepan
6. Stir well. Bring to a simmer and simmer covered for 10 minutes.
7. Strain and sweeten with honey to taste (if desired).

***Or buy Republic of Teas' Turmeric single sips (preblended pouches). However, by using fresh ingredients, you can adjust this recipe to taste and also take advantage of the wonderful scents as it simmers.*

Hummus with Vegetables

Ingredients
- 4 oz Hummus (purchase or use the recipe below)
- Sliced red/yellow/orange bell peppers
- Broccoli crowns

Take a moment to pick a plate or bowl that you enjoy looking at and arrange the veggies and hummus in a pleasing way. This is a simple snack but it can be lovely to look at, elevating those happy chemicals.

Homemade Hummus
- 1 can garbanzo beans (you can use cannellini as well)
- 2 tbsp lemon juice (adjust as needed)
- 2 garlic cloves
- 1 tbsp tahini
- 2 tbsp extra virgin olive oil
- Pinch of salt

Instructions
Drain and rinse the beans. Place all ingredients in a food processor and blend until smooth. You may need to add a bit of water or oil to thin the mixture. (Oil will create a stronger oil flavor.) Adjust salt and lemon juice to taste. Add other herbs/spices if you like (paprika, cumin, chili powder are all commonly used spices).

Happiness in a Bowl: Fruit Salad and Cheese

Ingredients
- Bananas
- Cantaloupe
- Oranges
- Strawberries
- 1/4 cup honey
- 1 tbsp lime juice

Cut the fruit into bite sized pieces (add other fruit if you like) and place together in a bowl. Blend the honey and lime juice in a small bowl and drizzle over the mixed fruit. Let set for a few minutes for all the juices and flavors to emerge.

Serve fruit over a bowl of cottage cheese, or with a couple slices of your favorite cheese (real cheeses - not velveeta). You can also try adding crumbled goat cheese and fresh basil to the fruit as an alternative. By the way, one cup of the fruit salad is one serving of your fruits and vegetables for the day.

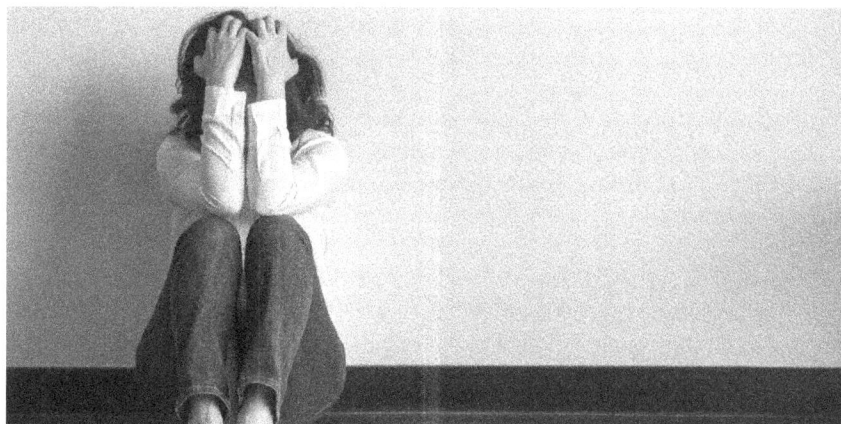

⊙ Anxiety/Anxiousness

Even though anxiety, or a sense of being anxious, feels like a strong emotion, there's actually a trigger (or triggers) for it. That trigger(s) is (are) the true emotion behind your feelings. Often anxiety is a consequence of suppressing guilt, shame, or fear. Frequently, it rises from an inability to express anger.(43)

If you suffer from anxiety, you are usually kind, polite, high-achieving, and self-critical. Anger is often not associated with your persona, yet it is present and buried beneath years of training it to "go away." Long ago, you likely learned that uncomfortable feelings, like anger, were not allowed to be expressed or validated. So those feelings became internalized. When anger is internalized rather than expressed, it can intensify the feeling of anxiety, leading to panic attacks and feelings of low self-worth.

Anxiety is a trickster that disrupts balanced eating habits. One day you feel fine and are making good health choices; the next day you don't want to leave the bed and aren't eating at all; the day after that, you are eating anything sugary; and the wheel keeps spinning.

For anxiety, practicing self-care is a priority with food being secondary. Eat antioxidant rich foods (much like a vegetarian) to nourish your body with necessary vitamins and minerals. One study by the National Institutes of Health showed that an anxious brain has lower levels of vitamins A, C and E.(44) So keep produce easily available at home and at work, but spend your energy on recognizing and using your tools to help you through the anxious feeling or moment.

Often anxiety can be relieved by one of the activities below. However, some anxiety issues become chronic, and you may need support from a medical doctor. If steps in this book are not helping, please talk to your doctor about further options.

To understand the foods and recipes that can help, refer to the "Anger," "Fear" and "Insecurity/Helplessness" Foods for Feelings sections. If you recognize another emotion behind the anxiety, refer to that section as well.

Chemical in charge: norepinephrine (low), serotonin (low), GABA (low)

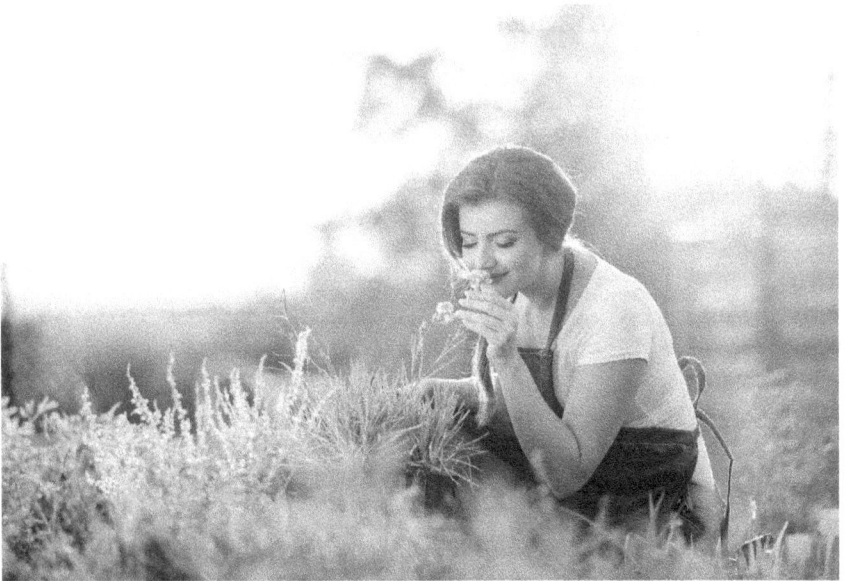

Activities that can help

- Practicing Mindfulness Meditation (see page 49)
- Listening to your favorite music
- Cleaning something
- Knitting or Crocheting
- Doing a jigsaw puzzle
- Gardening
- Doing something creative like painting or scrapbooking
- Aromatherapy
- Getting a good night's sleep (refer to the Sleep section see page 33)
- Practicing gratitude (refer to the Gratitude section see page 54)

Essential Oils

- Lavender or Chamomile
- Bergamot
- Rose

Exercises/movement that can help

- Going for a jog or run for at least 20 minutes
- Walking in nature (see page 42)
- Reverse lunges
- Clockwork lunges
- Jumping jacks

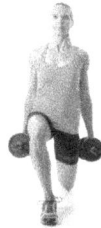

Reverse Lunge

Helpful Yoga poses

- Tortoise
- Savasana
- Warrior 2
- Child's Pose
- Seated Forward Fold
- Legs up the wall
- Down Dog

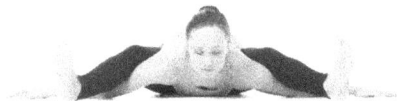

Tortoise Pose

Reflect and Journal

- When did/does your anxiety start?
- Is there a situation that causes your anxiety? Can you change the situation?
- What would an anxiety-free day/month look like for you? What steps can you take to make that your new reality?

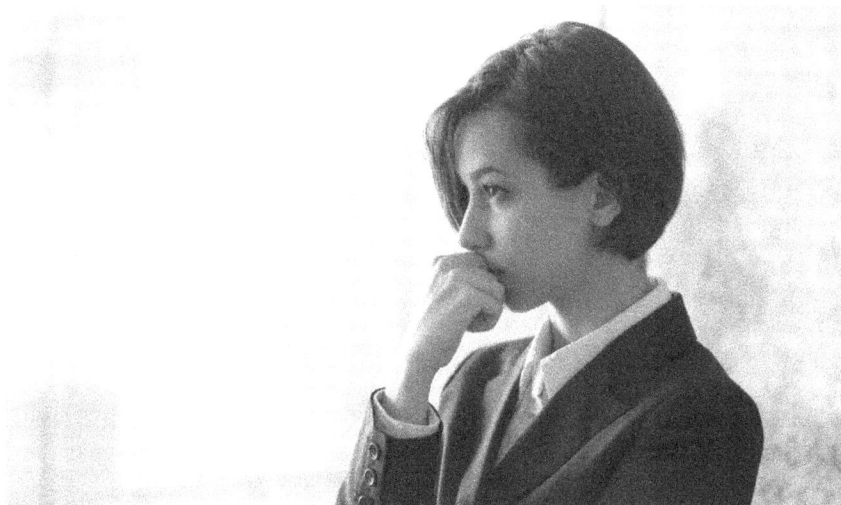

⊙ Insecure/Helpless

"I just can't deal anymore."

"I'm not a very good (insert mom, friend, employee here)."

"These jeans make me look fat."

Have you had these thoughts? We all have at one time or another, and they come from an emotion of insecurity or helplessness.

It is a feeling of being vulnerable. Being inferior. Being evaluated or judged. It comes from a fear of failing or rejection - or from actually failing or being rejected.

If you grew up with critical parents and friends, then you may be more sensitive to or concerned with how others perceive you, distorting your own beliefs about your self-worth and the idea that others are always evaluating you.

Feeling insecure or helpless can come from a need to be "perfect." When you don't meet that expectation, disappointment follows, leading to an insecurity that you are not enough. Not meeting perfection can mean constant - daily - disappointment. This can further lead to poor self-esteem and body image.

When you feel insecure or helpless, you may eat more, or you may start an extreme diet. Either way, focusing on food gives you a sense of being in control, even if it's misguided.

When you adopt a fad diet - or restriction diet - you are enforcing **control over your body**. You mentally decide the number of calories consumed and calculate the calories burned. You are likely obsessed with the number on the scale or size of your clothes. You know your body - you are not insecure.

When you overeat - or binge - you are taking **control over the food itself**. You have control over the shopping, cooking, eating - all giving you a sense of purpose and power. You are not helpless.

Unfortunately, being outwardly focused on your body or food and eating for reasons stemming from insecurity/helplessness means misinterpreting hunger cues and body satiation (fullness and satisfaction).(45) You truly are not aware of when you are hungry or not, full or not, or if you are even enjoying the food. Mindful Eating (see page 42) will help you in reclaiming your enjoyment of food, tuning in to your body's cues, and feeling more secure in your skin!

Chemicals in charge: oxytocin (too low), dopamine (too low), serotonin (too low/unbalanced)

Foods that can help

- Meat: all varieties, just keep the portion size to 4 ounces
- Fish: salmon, mackerel, tuna
- Eggs
- Green, leafy vegetables, especially spinach, chard, and kale
- Vegetables like peas, broccoli, cabbage, green beans, artichokes, asparagus, brussels sprouts, and potatoes
- Fruits like figs, banana, and raspberries
- Avocados
- Nuts and seeds such as pumpkin seeds, flaxseeds, almonds, walnuts, and cashews
- Beans, especially black beans, chickpeas, edamame, and kidney beans
- Yogurts
- Whole grains and quinoa
- Spirulina
- Dark chocolate

Activities that can help

- Sharing a meal - release oxytocin with your loved ones!
- Being flexible and keeping rational thoughts. You will have this emotion, how do you handle it?
- Taking action - do something, anything but eating, to feel less helpless. (For example, are you feeling helpless that the bees are dying? Donate money to programs that help and buy local honey.)
- Going to the movies with a friend
- Reading a book, especially one that is uplifting or happy
- Creating stability in life: take steps to fix any areas of uncertainty
- Hugging others
- Taking a warm bath with epsom salts
- Giving a gift or performing a random act of kindness
- Dancing and playing (like your a little kid again)
- Having sex (yep, this one's great for feeling body confident!)
- Crying, if you need to, and... then... taking action!

Essential Oils

- Jasmine
- Frankincense
- Sandalwood

Exercises/movement that can help

- Jump squats
- Reverse lunge with knee up
- Any movement that makes you feel empowered!

Jump Squat

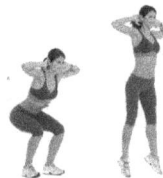

Helpful Yoga poses

- Tortoise
- Seated Forward Fold
- Side Plank
- Crow
- Child's pose
- Triangle
- Upward facing dog

Triangle Pose

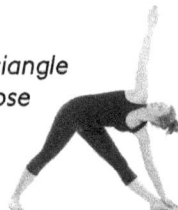

Healthy snack recipes

- Spirulina Energy Balls
- I Got This! Tuna Salad
- Quick Boost Egg and Chard
- Roasted Vegetables and Quinoa

Reflect and Journal

- When did your insecurity start? How old were you? What was the environment/situation?
- What does helplessness/insecurity feel like in your body?
- How does insecurity/helplessness drive you to eat?
- What non-food activities feel stable and reliable to you?
- What is the purpose of feeling helpless or insecure? Is there a lesson you can learn from this?
- Is your helplessness/insecurity learned or self-inflicted? Are you listening to your critical voice and not your true voice? How can you quiet the critical voice?
- Does your insecurity come from a lack of having certain skills? Can you learn these skills or ways to improve your confidence?

Recipes

Spirulina Energy Balls
(this recipe courtesy of and adapted from Copina Co.)

Ingredients
- 1 cup raw almonds
- 1 cup pitted dates (medjool are awesome, but use deglet and just soak them a bit if you don't have them)
- 1 lemon peel (add peel to taste and do not add lemon juice)
- 1 tbsp spirulina powder
- 1 tbsp cocoa powder (add more if desired)
- Shredded coconut (optional)

Instructions
Put nuts into a food processor and break them up first. Then add the rest of the ingredients. Process until smooth, then form into tiny balls. Roll in the coconut if desired. Keep them in your fridge in an airtight container for up to a week. Strain and sweeten with honey to taste (if desired).

I Got This! Tuna Salad

Ingredients
- 1 can (8 oz) Tuna in water, drained
- 1 celery stalk, diced
- 1 dill pickle, diced
- Pickle juice
- 1/2 green apple, diced (optional)
- 1/4 cup sliced almonds
- 1 tsp ground flaxseeds
- 1/2 cup raw spinach, or 1/4 shredded brussel sprouts
- 1/3 cup mayonnaise

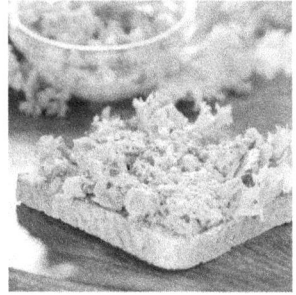

Instructions
Combine all ingredients in a bowl and mix well. Pour a splash of pickle juice and blend. Add salt and pepper to taste. Adjust other ingredients to your liking. Serve with whole grain, rice or nut crackers (see chicken salad recipe on page 63) or serve on a slice of toasted sourdough.

Quick Boost Egg and Chard

Ingredients
- 1 hardboiled egg
- 1/2 cup raspberries
- 2 cups sliced chard
- 1 tbsp olive oil
- Red wine vinegar
- Salt and pepper

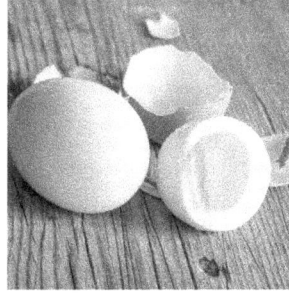

Instructions
Boil the egg until hard (about 8 minutes), then set aside to cool. While boiling, saute the chard in the olive oil. If you have garlic infused olive oil, even better! Once chard is wilted, turn off the heat and add a splash of red wine vinegar and a pinch of salt. (You can use lemon juice instead of the vinegar if you prefer.) Peel the egg and slice onto a plate. Sprinkle with salt and pepper. Place raspberries and chard on plate and enjoy.

**Alternately, you can also toast a piece of sourdough, layer with the chard and top with the egg. Serve with a side of raspberries. This makes a great breakfast as well!

Roasted Vegetables and Quinoa

Admittedly, this recipe isn't as much of a snack as a complete meal. However, I like to make it once, then eat it like a snack throughout the week.

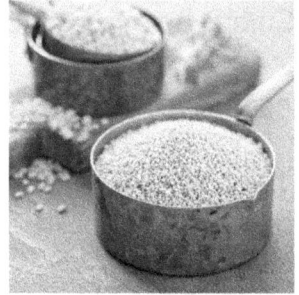

Ingredients
- 1 cup quinoa, rinsed and drained. (Follow cooking instructions)
- ~20 Brussel sprouts
- 1 sweet potato,
- 1/2 head of cauliflower
- 1 full stalk of broccoli
- 1/4 cup of pumpkin seeds
- Goat cheese (optional)

For the dressing:
- 1/3cup garlic infused olive oil
- 1/4 cup white wine vinegar
- 2 tsp apple cider vinegar
- 2 tbsp tahini
- 2 tsp lemon juice
- 2 tbsp maple syrup
- A bit of salt and pepper

Instructions
Chop veggies and place together in a bowl. Coat veggies with olive oil, salt and pepper, a dash of paprika and a dash of thyme. Roast veggies in a single layer on a baking sheet at 400 degrees for about 28 minutes or until nicely browned. When quinoa is done, put into a large bowl and let it cool. Once veggies are roasted, allow them to cool a bit as well. Once cooled, mix veggies into the quinoa, add the pumpkin seeds and cover with the dressing. Top with a bit of goat cheese if desired. Adjust the dressing to taste. Add a little more of this or that. The more tahini you use, the thicker the dressing as well.

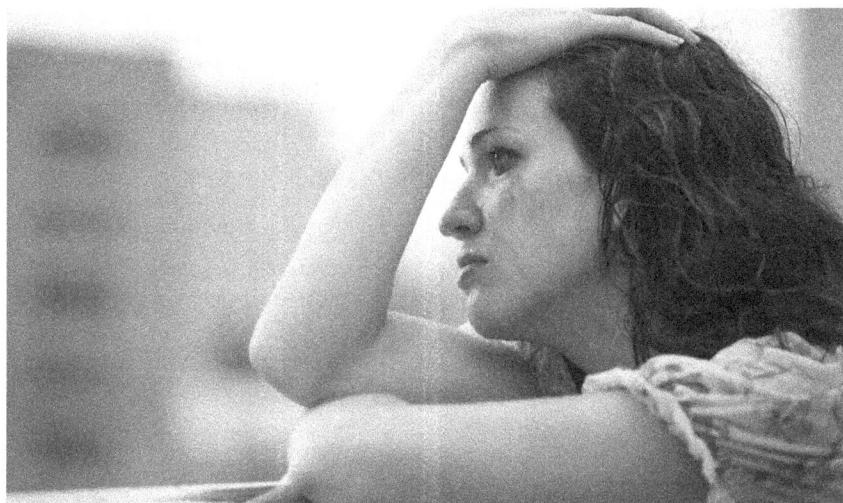

⊙ Sadness/Grief

I used to hate feeling sad until I realized that you cannot truly appreciate happiness until you've known sadness. They are yin/yang emotions, and sadness is inevitable. Sadness is a temporary state with many outlets to find relief. However, if you feel that your sadness is heavy and not going away, please refer to the chapter on "Depression" (see page 66).

Grief

Grief is overwhelming sadness. It can feel like it lasts forever, because, in some ways, it does. Grief occurs when we experience a profound loss. This could be the death of a loved one, end of a career, separation from a home, divorce, or more. Grief encompasses sadness, depression, insecurity, and fear of the unknown. But these things will heal with time and dedication to your improved well-being. Some grief exists deeply, and your love will just have to grow around it in a constant hug. Some grief will fade away as circumstances in life change.

It is common to lose your appetite when you are sad or grieving. If this is the case for you, pay close attention to the **Foundational Solutions** in this book and the activities below to help guide you towards more happiness and fulfillment.

85

Foods that can help

- Soy foods - quality tofu and edamame (not foods with soy protein isolate)
- Cheese, especially Parmesan, Gruyere, Swiss, and hard goat cheese
- Nuts, especially almond, peanut, walnut, cashew, and pistachio
- Seeds, especially pumpkin, sunflower, chia, sesame, and flax
- Meat - beef, lamb, chicken, pork, fish (especially tuna)
- Eggs - select pasture-raised for higher Omega-3 content
- Dairy, especially yogurt, buttermilk, and sour cream
- Beans - all kinds, but especially pinto beans
- Whole grains especially kamut, quinoa and wild rice
- Vitamin A rich foods and beta-carotenes: apricots, broccoli, cantaloupe, carrots, collard greens, peaches, pumpkin, spinach, and sweet potato
- Vitamin C rich foods: blueberries, broccoli, grapefruit, kiwi, oranges, peppers, potatoes, strawberries, and tomato
- Mushrooms
- Avocados
- Easy to digest foods if you are not hungry (eating still helps though)
  - Soups, smoothies, mashed potatoes, bananas, bone broth
- Minimize or avoid caffeine and alcohol
- Chamomile, peppermint, or green tea
- Dark chocolate

Activities that can help

- Listening to music (but not sad music unless you know that it helps)
- Watching a funny movie
- Spending time with friends (avoid isolation)
- **Crying!** Let the endorphins flow. Don't hold back the tears; it does not help you.

Essential Oils

- Bergamot
- Grapefruit or lemon
- Cedarwood or Cinnamon

Exercises/movement that can help

- Gentle Yoga
- Jump squats
- Jogging/walking
- Shoulder bridge

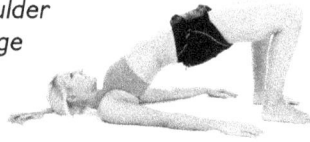

Shoulder Bridge

Helpful Yoga poses

- Child's Pose
- Standing Forward fold
- Pigeon
- Supine twist
- Legs up the wall
- Dancer

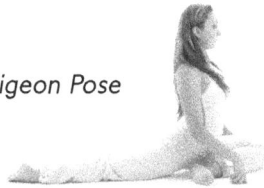

Pigeon Pose

Healthy snack recipes

- Edamame
- Roasted Parmesan Chickpeas
- Avocado Toast
- Toasty Goodness
- Berry Good Yogurt

Reflect and Journal

- What is the source of your sadness? Is it something that you can control or is it out of your control? Where can you influence positive change?
- How do you usually deal with feeling sad, lonely, or isolated? What are some ways for you to find emotional fulfillment and comfort besides eating?
- Does your sadness occur at the same time of day or day of the month? What is happening in that moment?
- Can you recognize what it feels like to sit **with** your grief rather than **in** it?

Recipes

Edemame

This couldn't be easier. Select the **unshelled variety** at the store (in the freezer section). The pods, or skins, tend to pick up more flavor than the beans alone. Also, the act of removing the bean from the pod is itself a mindful way of eating and connecting with your food and yourself.

Ingredients
- 1 cup of heated edamame (heat according to directions)
- Add a flavor combination:
  - Salt and rice vinegar (enough to lightly season and coat), garlic-infused olive oil and grated parmesan, chili powder and lime juice, or dash of soy sauce and ginger powder

Instructions
You can also try **roasted edamame** for a crunchy snack. Simply preheat the oven to 475 degrees. Thaw, rinse and dry the edamame and place in a bowl. Coat the beans with olive oil, salt and your choice of herbs and spices. Spread evenly on a baking sheet and roast for about 20 minutes (or until crispy but not burned), turning beans at the 10 minute mark.

Roasted Parmesam Chickpeas

For a long time, roasted chickpeas was my go-to snack. They are super easy and super cheap to make yourself. Just in case you need it - garbanzo beans and chickpeas are the same thing.

Ingredients
- 1 can of garbanzo beans, drained and rinsed
- 1 tbsp olive oil
- 1 garlic clove, minced (or use garlic powder to taste)
- 2 tbsp shredded parmesan cheese

Instructions
Preheat the oven to 400 degrees. Rinse the beans and lay evenly on a paper towel. Dry the beans thoroughly. It's OK if the outer skin comes off. Place beans in a bowl and mix with the other ingredients. Spread coated beans in a single layer on a baking sheet and roast for about 15 minutes. Turn the beans and roast for another 15 minutes or until golden brown and crispy. Cool and enjoy.

**These are best eaten within one or two days; then the beans begin to lose crispness.

Berry Good Yogurt

Ingredients
- 1 cup greek yogurt (avoid nonfat yogurts: you need fat to absorb calcium)
- 1 tsp raw, unfiltered honey
- 1/2 cup organic blueberries or strawberries (or both)
- 1/2 cup vanilla and nut granola (select your favorite low sugar variety)
- 1/2 tsp chia seeds

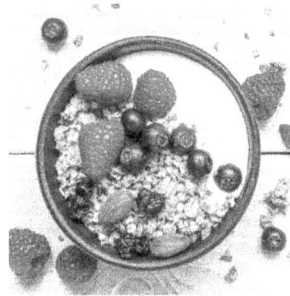

Instructions
Combine all ingredients in a bowl and enjoy!

Avocado Toast

Ingredients
- 1 slice of sourdough bread
  (or your favorite multi-grain bread)
- 1/4 to 1/2 avocado
- 1/2 tsp sesame seeds
  (or 1 tbsp pumpkin seeds)
- 1/2 cup arugula greens
- Sea salt
- 1 cup of strawberries

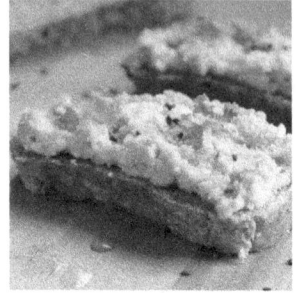

Instructions
Toast the bread in a toaster. Spread the avocado on the toast. Top with a sprinkle of sea salt, seeds and greens. Serve with strawberries on the side.

Avocado toast is a wonderfully basic and diverse snack. You can top the avocado with just about anything you like to make a snack or a meal. Try tomato or cucumber; cilantro, chili and lime; salmon and basil; olives or even an egg.

Toasty Goodness

Ingredients
- 1 slice of sourdough bread
- 2 oz of goat cheese
- 1/2 cup each of chard, kale and spinach
- 1/2 cup diced zucchini or yellow squash
- 1 tbsp olive oil
- Sea salt

Instructions
Sautee squash or zucchini in the olive oil until soft and set aside. (You may add garlic powder or other seasonings to the squash if you like.) Add the greens into the pan with more olive oil (if needed) and cook until gently wilted. While those are cooking down, toast the bread in a toaster and smooth a layer of goat cheese across the top. Top the cheese with the cooked squash followed by the wilted greens. Sprinkle with a dash of salt. Yum! *I often add a gently fried egg on top and turn this into a meal.*

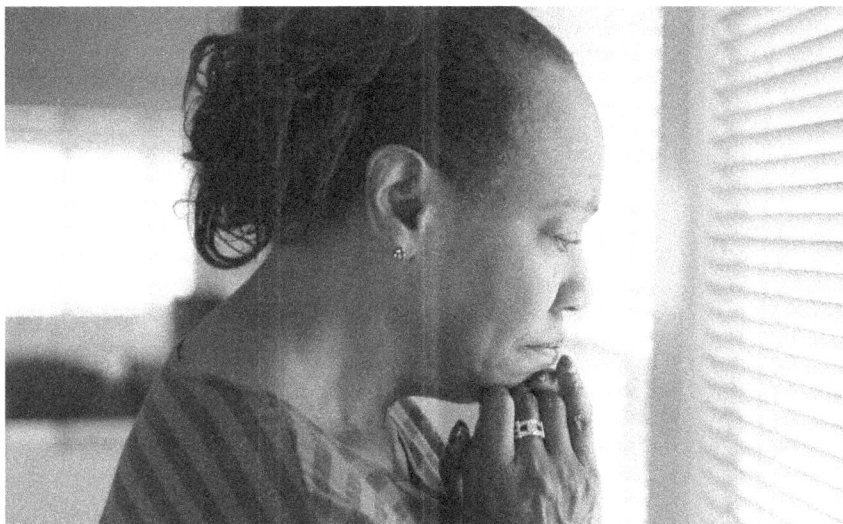

⊙ Fear

We don't often link our emotional eating with fear. After all, we aren't being chased by a bear, so what's there to be afraid of? But if you look at fear closely, you'll realize that it masquerades as other feelings: worry ("What if...?"), anxiety ("What's coming...?"), doubt ("I'm not good enough for..."), and indecision ("I'm not smart enough to...") to name several.

Fear can be immediate - "Don't step off the cliff!" - and then fade away once the danger passes. But emotional eating comes from a fear that is constant and nagging. This fear is triggered by memory; something that you learned in your past and associated a "fear" feeling with - be it a specific environment or activity. Did you get lost in the woods as a child? If so, you may feel fear just by smelling a pine scent. Memory is powerful and connected to areas in the brain that are also connected to emotions.

For fear, GABA plays a major role. Glutamate - the main chemical sensor between neurons and the precursor to GABA - allows GABA-mediated inhibition of fear to be exerted across the neural pathways.(46) Remember when I mentioned "neuro-plasticity" in the brain? Glutamate allows for flexibility in your response to fear.

This means that if you access your fear-inducing memory in a safe, "nonassociative" environment, then the memory will fade and be replaced with a safe feeling.(47) In contrast, if the memory is accessed in a setting that reaffirms the fear feeling, then it is strengthened.

So "facing your fears" is a valuable solution, but do it in a safe place!

So you know that GABA is highly involved, but other neurotransmitters also contribute to emotional eating around fear. Generally when you are fearful, you are less hungry but more inclined to eat impulsively.(48) You select comfort foods because they are dependable and there are no surprises. You know exactly what you are getting with pizza or ice cream, and your memory reminds you that it helps!

Chemicals in charge: GABA (too little), dopamine (too high), serotonin (too high/unbalanced)

Foods that can help

- Cheeses like Parmesan, cheddar, Swiss, and mozzarella
- Vegetables, especially tomatoes, corn, mushrooms, broccoli, potatoes, dark leafy greens, asparagus, and red bell peppers
- Avocados
- Fish like salmon, scallops, and shrimp
- Beef (3-4 ounce servings)
- Limit chicken and Turkey
- Limit eggs
- Beans
- Nuts and seeds, particularly pumpkin, sesame, peanuts, cashews, pistachios
- Grains, like wheat, barley, and oats
- Fruits, especially bananas, apples, grapes, and citrus
- Chamomile, matcha, or licorice teas
- Olive and coconut oils
- Minimize or avoid fermented foods (but only if you know they are a trigger for your fear state. Otherwise fermented foods could balance your microbiome to help with fear.)
- Reduce or avoid caffeine
- Avoid alcohol
- Avoid sodas and sugary drinks
- Avoid hydrogenated oils (think non-dairy creamers)

Activities that can help

- **Meditating and breathing** (see page 49): A process called potentiation amplifies your fear response if you are in a state of fear. (Every tickle on your skin makes you think it's a spider because one landed on your arm earlier.) Connecting with your breathing will stop this process.
- **Talking to a friend (or therapist)**: Vocalizing the fear externalizes it and helps to release it's hold on you.
- **Practicing being brave**: Sometimes you will have to do something that you are afraid of - giving a presentation at work, confronting a parent, interviewing for a job. Practice the activity with a person you trust until you feel confident and are no longer afraid.

Essential Oils

- Lavender
- Vetiver
- Clary Sage

Exercises/movement that can help

- Shadow boxing
- Russian twist
- Running/jogging/sprinting

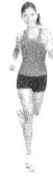

Helpful Yoga poses

- Crow
- Bow
- Forearm plank
- Pyramid
- Standing Big Toe

Forearm Plank

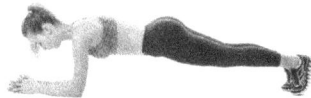

Healthy snack recipes

- Pumpkin Granola
- Salmon Treats
- Grilled Cheese and Tomato Soup
- Bean and Corn Salsa

Reflect and Journal

- What causes you to have a general feeling of fear? Why?
- What triggers your specific fears (if you have any)? Where were you? What did you see, hear, smell, or taste? Was it something a person said or did?
- Is the source a rational or irrational fear? Is this a new or chronic fear?
- What fear causes you to overeat, eat out of balance, or eat in an unhealthy way? How do you know?
- Can you avoid the fearful situation? If not, what is a safe place to confront your feelings? If yes, does avoidance solve the problem?
- What are some ways you can overcome this fear without food?

⊙ Recipes

Pumpkin Granola

(recipe courtesy of and adapted from Lindsay at her Pinch of Yum blog). I like the idea of this granola to calm fear, as the act of measuring, mixing, baking and smelling as it cooks tend to calm an overactive nervous system.

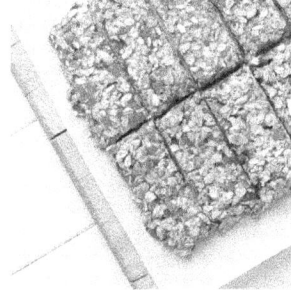

Ingredients
- 6 cups rolled oats
- 1 cup sliced almonds
- 1 cup pistachios
- 1 cups unsweetened flaked coconut
- 1 cup pumpkin puree
- 1 cup olive oil
- 1 cup maple syrup
- 1 to 2 tsps sea salt (more salt means more salty/sweet flavor)
- 1 to 2 tsps cinnamon
- 1/8 tsp fresh grated nutmeg
- 1/4 cup pumpkin seeds

Instructions
Preheat the oven to 350 degrees. Mix the dry ingredients together (except for the pumpkin seeds). Whisk the wet ingredients and spices together. Pour wet ingredients over the dry ingredients and combine. Spread the granola onto a nonstick baking pan and bake for 15 minutes. Add the pumpkin seeds, stir and bake for another 15 minutes. Remove from the oven and let it rest to crisp up. Store in an airtight container or plastic bag for about a week. Eat as is, or serve with yogurt and/or fruit.

Salmon Treats

Ingredients

- 1 package wild caught smoked salmon or lox
- Sliced swiss cheese
- Asparagus or fresh basil or spinach
- Olive tapenade (I prefer a greek olive blend.)
- Crackers

Instructions

Select about six of your favorite multi-grain, rice or nut crackers. Spread a layer of olive tapenade on top along with a bit of swiss cheese. (You may also decide one or the other, cheese vs. tapenade, instead of both.) Place a layer of salmon on top. Most varieties of lox come sliced already. Add a layer of raw or cooked asparagus, or basil or spinach to the top. If you are not using the tapenade, you may need a dash of sea salt as well. This makes a quick snack or meal, depending on how many crackers you decide to eat.

Bean and Corn Salsa

I like this recipe because it is so easy to make, super yummy, and can be made in a large batch to eat throughout the week. You can eat it as is, or add as a topping to salads, eggs, or tacos. *(recipe courtesy of Amy at The Blond Cook blog)*

Ingredients
- 1 (15-ounce) can yellow whole kernel corn, drained
- 1 (15-ounce) can black beans, drained and rinsed
- 1 cup chopped red onion
- 2 cups seeded and chopped roma tomatoes
- 1/3 cup seeded and chopped jalapenos
- 1/4 cup fresh chopped cilantro
- 1/4 cup lime juice
- 1/2 teaspoon cumin
- 2 tablespoons olive oil
- 1/2 teaspoon salt (more or less, to taste)
- 1/2 teaspoon pepper (more or less, to taste)
- Organic tortilla chips

Instructions
Place all ingredients (except tortilla chips) in a large bowl and stir to combine. Serve with tortilla chips. (A snack portion should be about 8 to 10 chips).

Grilled Cheese and Tomato Soup

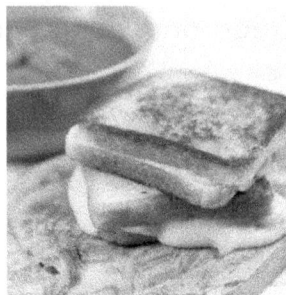

As I've said - let's keep this simple. If you have time to make a homemade tomato soup, awesome! If not, choose a canned soup with minimal added ingredients and/or sugar. Right now, I am enjoying the Simple Truth brand of tomato soup with organic tomatoes. Whenever possible, buy soups, sauces, and marinades made with organic tomatoes.

Ingredients
- 2 slices of sourdough bread
- 1 or 2 slices of sharp cheddar
- 1 or 2 slices of monterey jack
- 1 slice of pepper jack
- 1 slice of gruyere (optional)
- 1 can condensed tomato soup
- Milk
- Dried basil

Instructions
Place cheese between two slices of bread to make a sandwich. Spread a thin layer of mayonnaise on the outside of the bread and place in a pan over low to medium heat. Turn sandwich often to keep from burning and to allow for even melting. It is ready when it is golden and melty.

Pour soup into a pot and fill the can half with milk and half with water (this will make it a creamier soup). Pour liquid into the pot and whisk. Allow to heat over low to medium heat, careful not to let it burn.

Serve soup in a bowl with a sprinkle of dried basil and with the melted grilled cheese on the side.

***Certainly this is a meal. As a snack you could always do half of a sandwich of the grilled cheese, adding cooked broccoli, asparagus, or tomatoes inside. If you are in a huge hurry, skip the sandwich. Eat a 3 ounce serving of cubed cheese with tomato slices and a handful of grapes!*

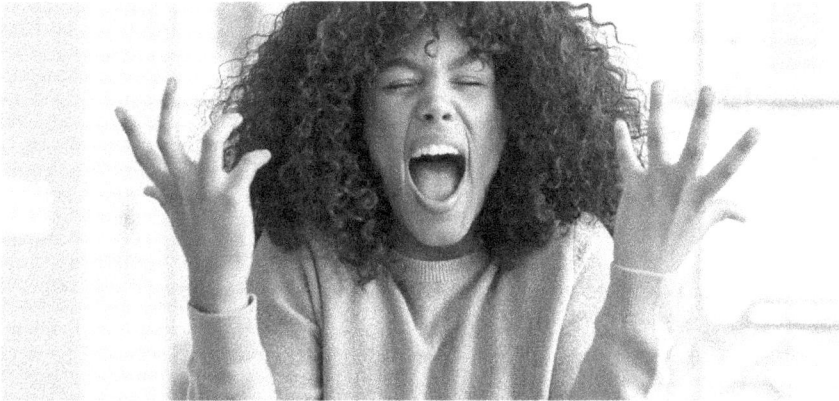

⊙ Anger

Are you an angry eater? I used to be. Now I'm an "angry cleaner." My house looks amazing when I'm mad! Eating when you're angry is actually pretty common. Very often, people who feel angry also feel an increase in hunger and have higher tendencies toward impulsive and sensory eating.(49)

Angry eaters may eat to avoid conflict (not get into a fight), or they may eat for "something to do" because they can't do anything about the situation at the time. Eating makes you feel better because you are **doing** something, in this case "angry chewing." Eating also gives you a way to take action while you decide on how ready you are to interact with people and your environment. It gives you a safe, and reliable, way to calm down.

Yet, swallowing your anger is a method of internalizing the struggle, hiding the frustration and slew of other emotions connected with your anger. You feel empty... and hungry... so now you are desperate to eat, desperate to no longer feel empty.

Angry eating is usually fast and mindless, which is a great way to overeat! You miss the taste of food and overlook your body's cues regarding hunger and fullness. I strongly suggest that you review the sections on "Mindful Eating" and "Meditation" to support your ability to manage anger when it attacks.

Chemicals in charge: acetylcholine (too high), GABA (too little), serotonin (too low), epinephrine (too much)

Foods that can help

Foods rich in the B vitamins are your best friend.
- Organ meats (like liver)
- Wild-harvested shrimp and clams
- Berries, especially blueberries
- Citrus, especially oranges
- Vegetables, specifically spinach, dark leafy greens, broccoli, yams, potatoes, tomatoes (choose cherry), brussels sprouts, asparagus, carrots, mushrooms and beets
- Apples
- Pears
- Avocados
- Beans, peas, and lentils
- Whole grains
- Olives and olive oil
- Herbs, specifically rosemary and ashwagandha (be careful with ashwagandha if you take thyroid medication and talk with your doctor).
- Fermented foods: Try the 4 "K's" - krout, kimchi, kefir, and kombucha.
- Yogurt, unsweetened (add a small amount of honey or berries)
- Chamomile, oolong, valerian, pu-erh, licorice, or green teas. Valerian is best used at night as it can promote sleep.
- Dark chocolate
- Sugar. Yep, it helps with anger, but choose wisely - a candy bar is not as helpful as an orange!
- **Minimize meats**: though a good source of B vitamins, eat lean or red meats in small portions (3 ounces). The tyrosine in meat helps with anger, but some of the other amino acids do not. This includes eggs.

Activities that can help

- **Showing loving-kindness to yourself**. Be accepting of your feelings and allow them to run their natural course. When anger arises, give yourself a hug and comfort the pain.
- **Breathing**. Pause and take deep breaths from the diaphragm to disengage from your "fight or flight" mode.
- **Writing it out**. You can do "angry writing" just as easily as "angry chewing." Getting your anger out on paper can be a good way to let the anger out rather than swallow it in. Often, putting words to your anger and acknowledging it is all you need.
- **Being prepared**: anger happens. Life will make you angry sometimes; it's unavoidable. Make a list, when you are calm and thoughtful, of things that you can do when you're angry that do not involve food.
- **Emptying your cupboards**. Keep processed foods, candy, and oily foods (potato chips) out of your house. If they are not available, then you can't eat them. And usually, you will not go out of your way to buy them. You will find a way to resolve your anger without emotionally eating.
- **Laughing**. Watch your favorite comedian on YouTube or turn on a comedy movie.
- **Talking it out**. Find a friend who can listen to and support you. Better yet, find someone who can make you laugh!

Essential Oils

- Lavender
- Bergamot
- Neroli

Exercises/movement that can help

- Boxing/Heavy bag work
- Burpees
- Jogging/running

Shadow Boxing

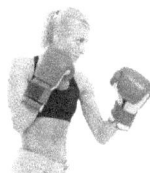

Helpful Yoga poses

- All twists
- Child's Pose
- Deep Breathing
- Back bends like Wheel or
  Upward Facing Dog

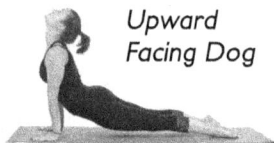

*Upward
Facing Dog*

Healthy snack recipes

- Quick shrimp scampi
- Spinach salad with fruit
- Loaded oats
- Kimchi fried rice

Reflect and Journal

- What is making you angry? Can you affect positive change?
- Is someone making you angry? Is there a way to make the relationship better? Does this person need to be in your life?
- In what ways can you better manage your anger?
- Are you struggling with a general sense of anger, or are you feeling a temporary anger?
- I notice that it's easier to choose foods mindfully, rather than automatically, when I...?

Shrimp Scampi

I know we don't usually think of shrimp as a snack. It's often saved for more "fancy" occasions. But shrimp takes very little time to cook and is easy to buy, so I think it deserves a place among "quick eats". Plus the sizzling sound is an added bonus when you are feeling angry.

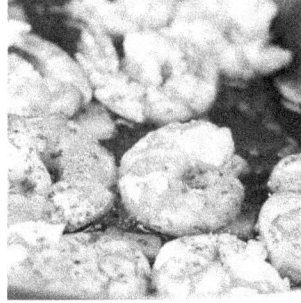

Ingredients
- Frozen, shelled shrimp (the amount that you would like for a snack; six maybe)
- 1 tbsp Olive oil
- 2 tbsp Unsalted Organic butter
- 1 to 2 garlic cloves, minced (or use garlic-infused oil)
- 1/8 to 1/4 cup dry white wine or chicken broth
- Salt and pepper
- Lemon juice
- Dried or fresh parsley

Instructions
Heat olive oil and half of the butter in a skillet. Add garlic and saute about a minute (do not let garlic burn). Add the shrimp and a pinch of salt and pepper. Cook shrimp for 1 to 2 minutes on each side (it should be slightly pink). Pour in the wine or broth and simmer for about 2 minutes. Add the remaining butter, lemon juice and a sprinkle of parsley and remove from the heat. Serve and enjoy! (Added bonus, throw some chopped broccoli, or other vegetables, in the remaining sauce and cook for a vegetable side.)

An even simpler version is to saute some shrimp in garlic-infused oil until cooked. Sprinkle with salt and pepper and enjoy. You can also buy fully cooked shrimp, thaw and eat as a shrimp cocktail with your favorite cocktail sauce. This version requires no cooking!

Spinach Salad with Fruit

Ingredients
- 1 to 2 cups of baby spinach
- 1/2 cup of arugula (optional)
- 1 clementine, peeled
- 1/2 pear sliced or diced
- 1/4 sliced red onion or 1 scallion
- 1/4 cup pecans
- 2 oz goat, feta or mozzarella cheese (optional)

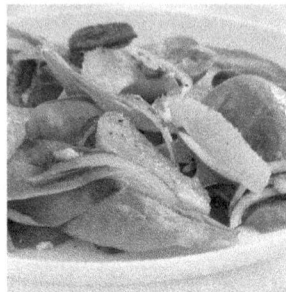

For the dressing
- 1 tbsp olive oil
- 1 tbsp apple cider vinegar
- 1 tsp dijon mustard
- 1 tsp honey
- 1/8 tsp dried rosemary
- Salt and pepper to taste

Instructions
Whisk together the ingredients for the dressing in a small bowl or measuring glass. Add more herbs, vinegar and/or honey to taste. More vinegar creates a vinaigrette. On a plate, top the greens with the fruit and nuts. Add cheese if you desire. Drizzle the dressing over the salad and serve. Keep any remaining dressing to use on other salads or roasted vegetables.

Loaded Oats

Ingredients
- 1 cup of steel cut oats
- ½ diced pear
- ¼ cup slivered almonds or walnuts
- Maple syrup

Instructions
Cook the oats according to the directions. Serve a snack or meal size portion and top with pear and nuts. Drizzle with maple syrup to your desired level of sweetness. **I prefer to make the overnight oats, so the oats are ready to heat and serve in the morning.*

Kimchi Fried Rice

This is definitely a meal, but I enjoy making a large amount and then eating leftovers as a snack or a quick lunch. Kimchi is available in jars in the fresh foods section in most grocery stores. This is a quick and tasty way to use leftover rice too!
**(recipe courtesy and adapted from of Anjali Prasertong via The Kitchn blog)*

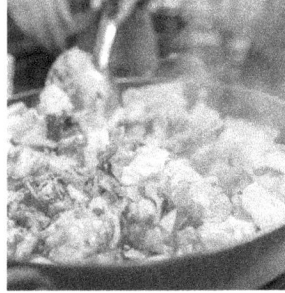

Ingredients
- 2 tbsp avocado or canola oil
- 1 cup cabbage kimchi, drained and coarsely chopped
- 1 tsp gochujang or sriracha
- 2 cups cold cooked white or brown rice
- 2 cups thinly sliced greens such as baby bok choy, kale, spinach, or Swiss chard
- 4 medium scallions, thinly sliced
- 1 to 2 tsp tamari or soy sauce
- 2 large eggs, lightly beaten (optional, start with one egg)
- 12 to 15 large shrimp, thawed, shelled and deveined
- 1/2 tsp Asian toasted sesame oil

Instructions
Heat the oil in a large skillet (cast iron is best or use a wok) over medium heat. Add the kimchi and gochujang or sriracha and stir-fry until hot, about one minute. Add the rice and cook another two minutes. Add the greens, scallions, and tamari or soy sauce. Stir-fry until the greens are cooked down and wilted. Taste and add more sauce if needed.

Push the rice to the side and pour in the egg in the empty space (optional). Stir and scramble the egg into soft curds. Mix the egg into the rice. Push the mixture to the sides, add a bit more oil in the empty space if needed and place the shrimp to cook. Cook about 2 minutes on each side until pink. Do not overcook. Mix the rice and shrimp together. Turn off the heat. Drizzle with the sesame oil (a little goes a long way), mix and serve.

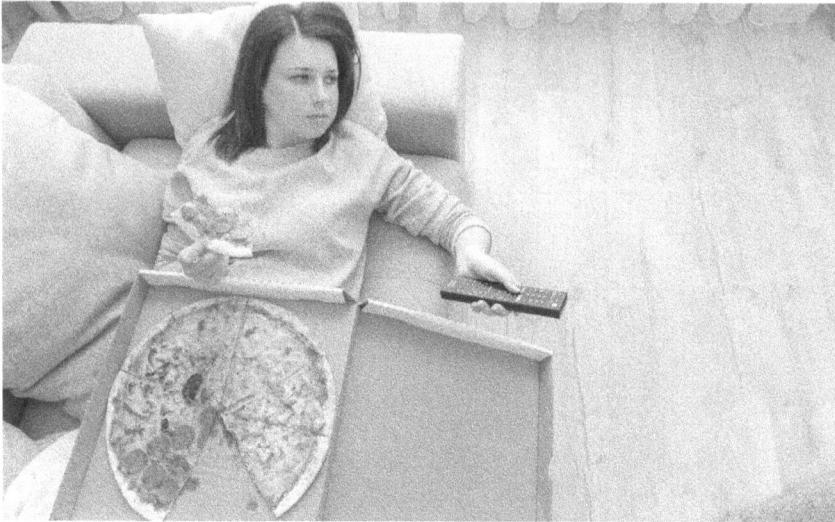

⊙ Laziness

"I'm just too lazy to take care of myself, I guess" - have these words crossed your mind or even your lips?

Laziness may feel like an emotion because it is an overall lack of vigor or enthusiasm. The drive and energy to do anything is lacking. But "lazy" isn't actually an emotion. It's more of a habit and is mostly a condition that is connected to feelings of apathy, fear, hopelessness, and a disconnection from the "self."

At best, feeling lazy is simply a state of being tired or overwhelmed. At worst, feeling lazy is a state of being deeply depressed. We all go through phases of laziness, especially if we have been constantly "on the go" and need a break, then we feel like "being lazy."

Laziness is different from procrastination though. Usually when you are lazy, you don't really know what you want to do or should be doing... or you really just need a break. With procrastination, you are very clear on what you need to and should do, you just want to avoid doing it.

With emotional eating, laziness appears as an inability to care for yourself. Strong feelings of apathy - "I just don't care" - cause you to reach for your favorite comfort foods (ice cream, a bag of chips, chips and queso). If the apathy stays with you while you're eating, there is a high chance that you will overeat that food. Then, as you reflect on what just happened, laziness makes you feel helpless... like you can't do anything to change. But you can! Listen to your inner guide and take one small step to get moving in a positive direction. "Lazy" can't keep up with a person on the move!

To understand the **foods and recipes** *that can help, refer to the "Fear" and "Insecure/helpless" Foods for Feelings sections.*

Chemicals in charge: happiness chemicals, especially dopamine (low) and GABA (low)

Activities that can help

- **Not skipping meals**. Drops in blood sugar can lead to a need for laziness.
- **Tracking your time**. Write down how you spend your hours. Perhaps you are already accomplishing a lot in a day and need down time. Or perhaps you are wasting time in non-productive ways which further endorse your idea of being lazy.
- **Setting realistic expectations**. Are you just expecting too much from yourself?
- **Identifying your life purpose** - without it, you are not driven by anything (like a car without an engine).
- **Setting a goal to do one thing differently** - start to break your habit!
- **Visualizing your "best self" as you meditate**. If you see yourself as active and motivated, you will begin to become that self (with a little work to break the habit).
- **Watching TedTalks** about motivation for inspiration.
- **Being social**: make a point to get yourself moving and out of the house.

Essential Oils

- Basil or Black Pepper
- Peppermint

Exercises/movement that can help

- Walking! (Refer to the walking section on page 40)
- Push ups
- Arm circles

Push Ups

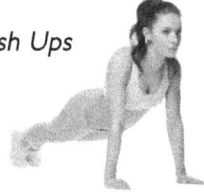

Helpful Yoga poses

- Frog
- Half Moon
- Sugarcane (Chapasana)
- Dancer
- Horse Squat
- Revolved Triangle
- Swan

Frog Pose

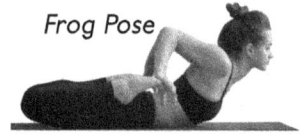

Reflect and Journal

- Evaluate - are you actually lazy or just comfortable with a slower pace of life?
- What used to get you excited and moving? Can you add more of that into your day?
- What is your life purpose? What feeds your fire to get up and get going?
- Do you know your personal values - what matters most to you? Can you name them with three words (for example: family, integrity, trust)? Are you living your values?
- How can you care for yourself? How can you "love you" every day?

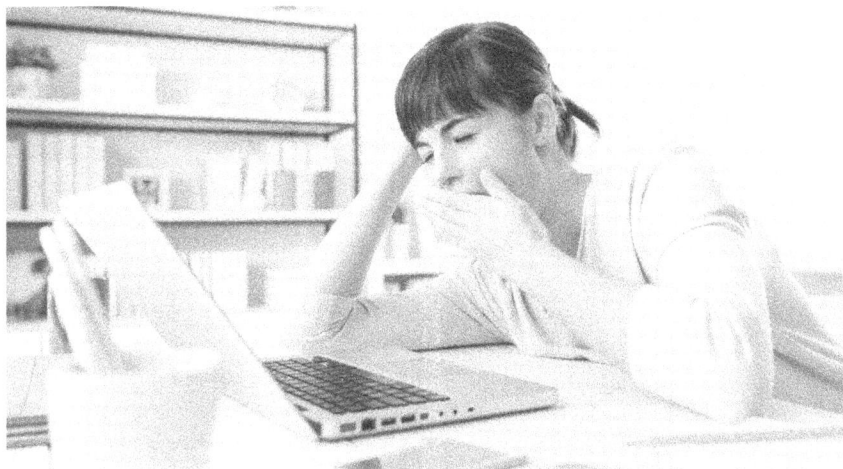

⊙ Tired

Feeling tired is right at the top with feeling bored when listed as why people eat emotionally. "I feel tired" is used so frequently in conversation that it should be an emotion. But again, tired isn't actually an emotion. It is fatigue or exhaustion, either physical or *emotional*.

Being physically tired can be due to many reasons:
- You ran a marathon!
- You didn't eat enough food.
- You worked long hours.

Being emotionally tired could be that:
- You had to make too many decisions (brain drain).
- You had events happen that brought up emotions.
- You cared for everyone but yourself.

What makes feeling tired a difficult problem is that being tired can create an emotion: "I'm so tired I just want to cry." Or the emotion can make you tired: "I cried so hard I'm tired."

Tiredness can also lead to emotional eating because you lack the enthusiasm to prep and cook a healthy, balanced meal. You are tired, so you grab whatever is available and eat. And since you are looking for energy, it is often something with sugar or simple carbs.

So, what should you eat when tired? Anything that nourishes you! Whole fruits and vegetables (especially leafy greens), seeds, lean meats, and dark chocolate (in small amounts). Carbohydrates (even complex carbs) will give you an increase in glucose, which will better energize you but don't overdo it. Eat just enough to keep you balanced, erase brain fog, and give you a dose of "pick me up." Foods rich in Omega-3 fatty acids can boost your drive and brain energy. These include salmon, avocado, flax seeds, hemp seeds, and pasture-raised meat.

You also will benefit from reducing or eliminating caffeine. I know, that seems wrong... caffeine wakes you up,right! But regular use of caffeine blocks adenosine (a sleep/wake hormone) in the brain, restricting this hormone from doing its job.(51) When adenosine binds to its receptors, you feel tired or sleepy. Caffeine doesn't stop it's production in the body, only its influence on the brain and the central nervous system. So when you stop drinking coffee or your energy drink, or even black tea, your brain floods with adenosine and you feel very tired! So use caffeine wisely - drink your coffee in the morning and trail off after 2pm. Or wean yourself slowly from caffeine by switching to Yerba Mate or Guayusa teas, and then down to green tea. The antioxidants in each will do your brain even more good!

To understand more specific **foods and recipes** *that can help, first identify the emotion connected with being tired, then refer to that Foods for Feelings section.*

Chemicals in charge: dopamine, GABA, norepinephrine, cortisol, melatonin (sleep hormone) - all out of sync

Activities that can help

- Not skipping meals, especially breakfast. Drops in blood sugar can lead to fatigue.
- Planning your meals and snacks. Make sure that you have healthy food available in the house, your car, your purse/bag. Don't fall victim to the "I'm tired so let's just go through the drive through" trap.
- Refer to the Sleep section (page 33)
- Refer to the Hydration section (page 37)
- Refer to the Meditation section (page 49)

Essential Oils

- To energize: peppermint, rosemary, eucalyptus
- To sleep: lavender, chamomile, vetiver

Exercises/movement that can help

- Moving can boost your energy, but start slow and gentle - yoga, general stretching, walking. Exercising too hard when your body is already tired can cause further imbalances with your brain chemistry and energy levels.
- When you are ready to get energy flowing try:
  - Jump rope
  - Bicycle crunches
  - Plank

Bicycle Crunch

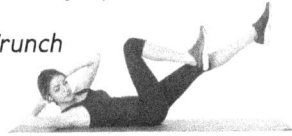

Helpful Yoga poses

- Headstand
- Shoulder stand
- Seated forward fold
- Inclined Plank
- Downward dog
- Camel
- Half lord of the fishes
- Crow squat
- Savasana

Half lord of the fishes pose

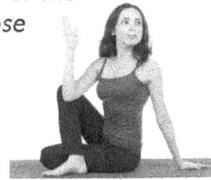

Reflect and Journal

- Evaluate - is your life unnecessarily burdened or overscheduled? Can you plan ahead to ease the burden, leaving you with more energy?
- Are you physically or emotionally tired? Why?
- Are you getting enough sleep?
- Are you eating enough calories to fuel your day?
- How is your overall health? Could your fatigue be caused by an underlying health issue (hypothyroidism, food/seasonal allergies, sleep apnea, diabetes for example)?
- Is there a person or situation that is an energy drain for you? What are some ways in which you can protect your energy from this person or situation?

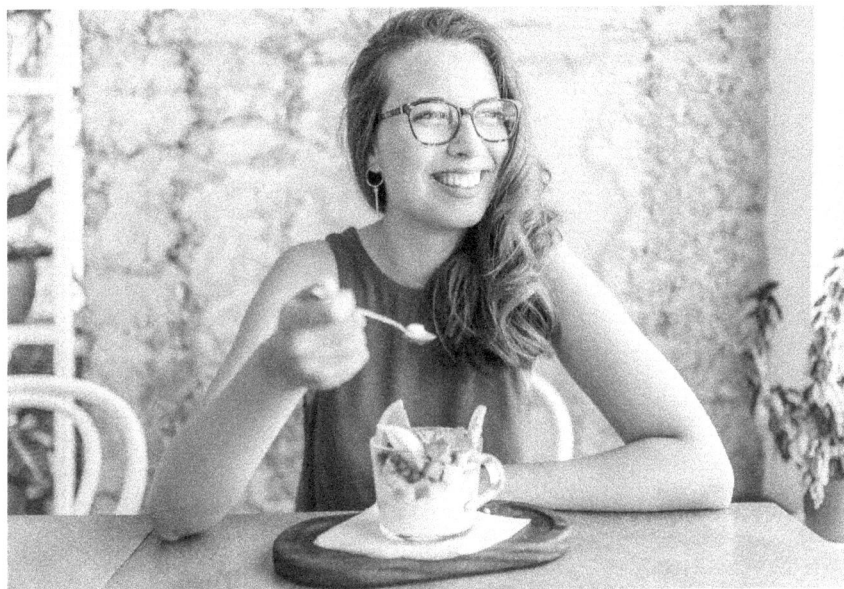

⊙ Reward

Food makes an excellent reward. Not only does it satisfy your brain (with dopamine), but it entices all your senses. For example, if you eat ice cream, you get a smooth texture, cold chill, sweet sugar, crunchy nuts or candy, and the pleasant smell of chocolate, mint, or vanilla. It's an engaging - and rewarding - experience.

As an emotion, reward is triggered by dopamine, which says, "Hey, you aced that exam, you deserve an ice cream!" Or, "Nice job cleaning the whole house, let's go out for dinner." Overall, we are very good at justifying our desire to eat by calling it a reward.

Reward can go both ways: We want a food, so we search for a reason to have it; or we have a reason to feel rewarded, so we seek out the perfect food. Sometimes feeling rewarded by a certain food results from conditioning. Consider the famous research of Ivan Pavlov and his dogs. You likely remember that Pavlov's dogs salivated when food was presented paired with the sound of bells. Over time, the dogs salivated simply from hearing the sound of a bell even when no food was presented. This is a conditional reflex brought about by conditioned stimuli.

Foods for Feelings

Humans are not very different from Pavlov's dogs when it comes to learning a conditional reflex. The stimuli we experience have the ability to activate complex emotional and motivational states in our bodies, and we want the reward that follows!(52) New research shows that dopamine is involved in *encoding memories about a reward* (how to get it, where it was obtained) and attributing importance to environmental stimuli that are associated with the reward.(53) In other words, when your bell sounds, you'll seek a reward in food.

The conditioning begins early. Often parents use food as a reward to achieve a desired behavior from their kids. "Eat your veggies, and you'll get dessert," or "Stop crying please, and I'll give you the cookie." So when we grow into adults, we are conditioned to have dessert after our salad!

Often reward is related to happiness. Afterall, you did a good job worthy of a reward! Refer to the Happiness section for more information on eating when you're happy. And while you may have been conditioned to reward yourself with food, you can retrain your brain! Earlier we talked about neuroplasticity and your brain's desire to learn and to create, so give your brain something to ponder - how can you reward yourself without food? What is the new reward waiting for you?

Chemicals in charge: dopamine (high), serotonin, oxytocin (elevated)

Foods that can help

Any foods/recipes in this book!
- Eat your "reward" food but do so mindfully (see page 42) and be certain that eating for reward remains a "sometimes" thing.
- Allow your "reward" food during normal meals, so that it's not related to a sense of being "rewarded." If your reward is always chocolate ice cream, then allow yourself a small bowl on a random day of the week. Begin to see it as just another food and not a reward. (Or, begin to retrain your brain.)
- Choose to reward your body with high quality nutrients rather than sugar, salt, or fat! Try replacement foods such as:
  - Yogurt with honey instead of ice cream
  - Roasted vegetables instead of french fries
  - Crunchy nuts or produce (carrots, apples) instead of chips
  - Quality cheese and crackers instead of Goldfish or cheesecake

Activities that can help

- **Doing any activity** that does not involve food but feels rewarding to you.
- **Buying an item** that you have been deeply wanting.
- **Sharing your story**. Talking through your excitement with others brings a reward through trust and bonding.

Essential Oils

- To calm the seaking mind: lavender or spearmint
- To bring contentment: patchouli or rose
- To feel rewarded: your favorite scent

Exercises/movement that can help

- **Any movement**. Getting your blood flowing further releases happiness hormones, including GABA, which makes you feel at peace or rewarded and content.
- Choose an exercise that you really enjoy to be rewarded without food: "I finished my chores, now I'm off for a bike ride!"

Helpful Yoga poses

- Side Moon
- Pigeon
- Down Dog
- Happy Baby
- Supine Butterfly
- Reverse Warrior
- Reverse Triangle
- Crow

Reverse Warrior

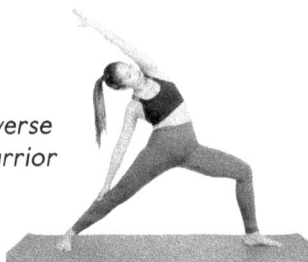

Reflect and Journal

- What is a "reward" food that you would like to learn to eat mindfully?
- Why do you use food as a reward?
- Are there other ways you can reward yourself?
- Is your need for a reward actually an excuse to eat? Is it an excuse to avoid feeling emotions?

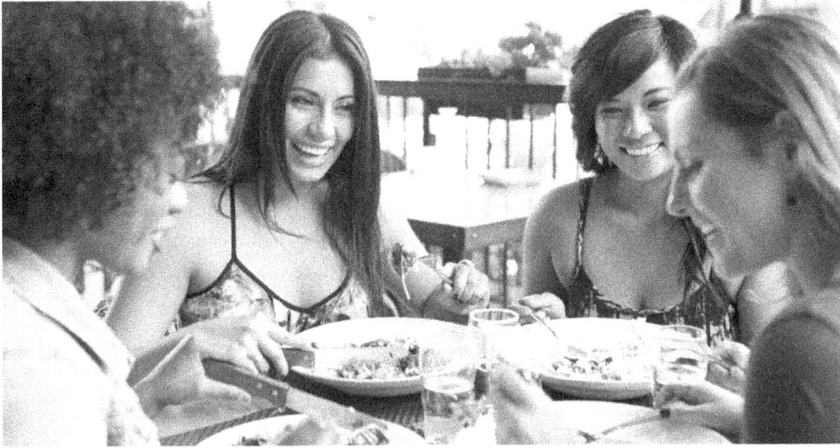

⊙ Happy

Eat and be happy! Or is it be happy and eat?

A friend recently told me, "I just eat, Amber. I eat when I'm sad. I eat when I'm happy." She said this as if it was a bad thing... like there's only one good time to eat, and she was doing it wrong.

Emotional eating means eating our emotions, and yes, that includes when we feel "happy." Studies have recently shown that emotional eaters actually consume more food due to positive moods compared to negative moods. *(50)*

And how could we not - happiness means celebration. And celebrations mean food! We eat for weddings, birthdays, promotions, graduations, anniversaries... The list goes on and on.

Major, wonderful life events all have food in common. This started with your very first birthday cake! *(Sadly, I was the uber-health mom, and my first son's cake was a carrot cake made with applesauce and a little low-sugar cream cheese frosting. Poor kid!)* Remember, we talked about "learned behavior." As early as one-year-old, you began connecting food with happy. And usually sweet and/or fatty food with happy!

Being in a happy mindframe also increases a desire for social interaction. You spend more time with friends and family, usually meeting them out for... **food**. Socially engaging usually means meeting at restaurants or coffee shops, which encourages eating.

Now celebrating and enjoying special occasions are a must. And eating for happiness only becomes a problem when you eat out of control or out of balance *each and every time you are happy*. "Oh, I'm so happy for you" (eat a Snickers); "Oh, this movie always makes me happy" (eat a large bag of popcorn); "Oh, the trees are so lovely. I'm so happy today" (drink a 40 ounce soda).

If you notice weight gain, health issues, or occasional feelings of guilt but you're generally a happy, easy-going person, then consider "happiness" as an emotional eating trigger. Pay attention to what you eat and in what quantity and commit to making some small changes to eat for the benefit of your body. Be happy... and stay happy!

Chemicals in charge: dopamine, serotonin, oxytocin (all three at elevated and balanced levels), as well as endorphins, adrenaline, GABA (all balanced)

Foods that can help

Any foods/recipes in this book!
- Your favorite foods, but eat mindfully (see page 42). Tune into your body and only eat if you are hungry (not because you are happy/celebrating).
- Vegetables and fruits with a little protein to keep the "happy" chemicals and your blood sugar in balance and steady. **It's easiest to make healthy food choices when you are happy, so fill your body with nutrient dense foods!**

Activities that can help

- Socializing with friends, but select a place or an activity that does not center around food (hiking, biking, etc.)
- Taking in some culture at an art or science museum
- Visiting a favorite location: botanic gardens, lake, store
- Trying a new hobby: fishing, archery, painting
- Listening to your favorite music or podcast

⬤ Essential Oils

- Geranium
- Grapefruit or Orange

⬤ Exercises/movement that can help

- Dancing
- Anything! What's your favorite movement?
- Chest fly - opening the heart space to the world. Use dumbbells (or cans of beans if needed).

Chest Fly

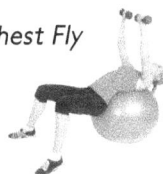

⬤ Helpful Yoga poses

- Headstand
- Shoulder stand
- Blossoming lotus
- Seated forward fold
- Camel

Shoulder Stand

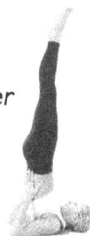

⬤ Reflect and Journal

- Why are you happy? Can you create more of that in your life daily?
- Who regularly makes you happy? In what ways can you connect with this person frequently?
- What challenges are present when you eat a meal with your family or friends? What makes social eating easier? What makes it harder?
- When you're happy, can you find ways to share that feeling with others?

Final Food
for Thought

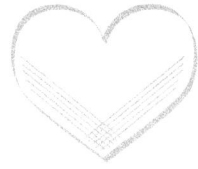

Emotions are complicated. They can be your best friend or your worst enemy... all in the same day. But emotions make you, well - YOU. Thanks to this book, you now have the knowledge and tools to be a happier, more balanced you. Food does not control you. Emotions do not decide what's for dinner. You are an aware individual eating and living mindfully.

It is my hope that you can find a nourishing and lovely relationship with food; that you can slow down and embrace food as a necessary and wonderful part of your day (rather than an afterthought as you pull through the drive-through).

At times, your emotions may feel like a burden or an immovable weight. You may feel trapped or constricted by your emotional eating. But I am here to tell you:

You were never designed to be bound by your body.

You are enough.

You are so much more.

You are bigger than life!

You are boundless!

References

1. Queensland Brain Institute. "What are neurotransmitters?" The University of Queensland, Australia, 9 Nov. 2017. Web.

2. Lakna. "Difference Between Hormones and Neurotransmitters." PEDIAA. 2 Jun 2017. Web.

3. Nanda, Aashish. "Hormones and Chemicals that Influence emotions." 2019. Web.

4. Brizendine, Louann. "The Female Brain." Pg 72. 2006.

5. Lieberstein, Andrea. Mindfulness-Based Eating Awareness Training and Coaching. 2016.

6. Hokuma. "Plutchik's Wheel of Emotions: What is it and HOw to Use it in Counseling." Positive Psychology Program. 24 Dec 2017. Web.

7. Henshaw, John M. "How many senses do we have?". John Hopkins University Press blog. 1 Feb 2012. Web.

8. Mergenthaler, Philipp; Lindauer, Ute; Dienel, Gerald A.; Meisel, Andreas. "Sugar for the brain: the role of glucose in physiological and pathological brain function." US National Library of Medicine National Institutes of Health. 20 Aug 2013. Web.

9. Bakalar, Nicholas. "Fructose May Increase Cravings for High-Calorie Foods." The New York Times. 4 May 2015. Web.

10. Luo, Shan; Monterosso, John R.; Sarpelleh, Kayan; Page, Kathleen A. "Differential
effects of fructose versus glucose on brain and appetitive responses to food cues and decisions for food rewards." PNAS. 19 May 2015. Web.

11. Anderson, Scott C. The Psychobiotic Revolution. Mood, Food and the New Science of the Gut-Brain Connection. Pg. 116. 7 Nov 2017.

12. Anderson, Scott C. The Psychobiotic Revolution. Mood, Food and the New Science of the Gut-Brain Connection. Pg. 121, 128. 7 Nov 2017.

13. Anderson, Scott C. The Psychobiotic Revolution. Mood, Food and the New Science of the Gut-Brain Connection. Pg. 56, 57. 7 Nov 2017.

14. Schneiderman, Neil; Ironson, Gail; Siegel, Scott D. "Stress and Health: Psychological, Behavioral, and Biological Determinants." US National Library of Medicine National Institutes of Health. 16 Oct 2008. Web.

15. Yau, Yvonne H. C.; Potenza, Marc N. "Stress and Eating Behaviors." US National Library of Medicine National Institutes of Health. 30 Oct 2014. Web.

16. Newman, E; O'Connor, D.B; Conner, M. "Daily Hassles and Eating Behaviour: The role of cortisol reactivity status." Psychoneuroendocrinology. PubMed. Pg. 125-32. PubMed. Web.

17. National Hearth, Lung and Blood Institute. "Sleep Deprivation and Deficiency." U.S. Department of Health and Human Services. 2018. Web.

18. Kahn, Michal; Sheppes, Gal; Sadeh, Avi; " Sleep and emotions: Bidirectional links and underlying mechanisms." International Journal of Psychophysiology. 24 May 2013. Article.

19. Merrell, Woodson. "Sleep More, Burn More Fat." Psychology Today blog. 14 Oct 2010. Web.

20. Harvard Health Publishing. "Vitamin D and your health: Breaking old rules, raising new hopes." Harvard Medical School. Feb 2007. Web.

21. Greenblatt, James M. "Psychological Consequences of Vitamin D Deficiency." Psychology Today blog. 14 Nov 2011. Web.

22. Patrick RP; Ames BN. "Vitamin D hormone regulates serotonin synthesis. Part 1: relevance for autism." US National Library of Medicine National Institutes of Health. 20 Feb 2014. Web.

23. Cooley, Jami. "10 Vitamin D Deficiency Symptoms You Can Identify Yourself. Fatigue, joint pain, low bone density, and weight gain: These and other ailments could be vitamin D deficiency symptoms that you can treat and even reverse." University Health News Daily. 28 Sep 2018. Web.

References

24. Lin, Steven. "Vitamin D Through Sun: 9 Tips to Optimize Your Levels." Dr. Steven Lin blog. 2018. Web.

25. Riebl, Shaun K.; Davy, Branda M. "The Hydration Equation: Update on Water Balance and Cognitive Performance." US National Library of Medicine National Institutes of Health. 1 Nov 2014. Web.

26. Field, T.; Hernandez-Reif, M; Diego, M; Schanberg S; Kuhn C. "Cortisol Decreases and serotonin and dopamine increase following massage therapy." US National Library of Medicine National Institutes of Health. Oct 2005. Web.

27. Hector. "Movement". ND Health Facts wiki. 13 Mar 2014. Web.

28. Chi-Jung Chen; Fang-Hua Chu; Shih-Chang Chien; Nai-Wen Tsao; Sheng-Yang Wang. "Comparative Analysis of Phytoncides Released from Liquidambar formosana Hance Trees and Seedlings." J. Agri. & Fore. Pg. 137-144. 18 Jun 2013. Article.

29. Shinrin-yoku Organization. "Go to a Forest. Walk slowly. Breathe. Open all your senses. This is the healing way of Shinrin-yoku Forest Therapy, the medicine of simply being in the forest." Shinrin-yoku blog. 2018. Web.

30. Lieberstein, Andrea. Mindfulness-Based Eating Awareness Training and Coaching. 2016.

31. Spence, Charles. "Just how much of what we taste derives from the sense of smell?". BioMed Central blog. 2 Nov 2015. Web.

32. National Institute on Deafness and other Communication Disorders (NIDCD). "Quick Statistics About Taste and Smell." US Department of Health and Human Services. 19 Oct 2018. Web.

33. Alankar, Shrivastava. "A Review on Peppermint Oil." Asian Journal of Pharmaceutical and Clinical Research. Volume 2, Issue 2, April- June, 2009. Pg 27-31. Article.

34. Fredrickson, B. L.; Cohn, M. A.; Coffey, K. A.; Pek, J.; Finkel, S. M. "Open hearts build lives: Positive emotions, induced through loving-kindness meditation, build consequential personal resources." Journal of Personality and Social Psychology, 95(5), 1045-1062. 2008. Article.

35. Davidson, Richard J. PhD; Kabat-Zinn, Jon PhD; Schumacher, Jessica MS; Rosenkranz, Melissa BA; Muller, Daniel MD, PhD; Santorelli, Saki F. EdD; Urbanowski, Ferris MA; Harrington, Anne PhD; Bonus, Katherine MA; Sheridan, John F. PhD. "Alterations in Brain and Immune Function Produced by Mindfulness Meditation." Psychosomatic Medicine: July 2003 - Volume 65 - Issue 4. Pg 564-570.

37. Miller, John J.; Fletcher, Ken.; Kabat-Zinn, Jon. "Three-year follow-up and clinical implications of a mindfulness meditation-based stress reduction intervention in the treatment of anxiety disorders." General Hospital Psychiatry: Volume 17, Issue 3, Pages 192-200. May 1995.

37. Greenberg, Melanie. "How Gratitude Leads to a Happier LIfe." Psychology Today blog. 22 Nov 2015. Web.

38. Roszak Burton, Linda. The Neuroscience of Gratitude: What you need to know about the new neural knowledge." *Wharton Healthcare Quarterly.* Oct 2016. Web.

39. Cespedes, Andrea. "Are There Foods That Cause the Release of Norepinephrine and Dopamine?" Livestrong blog. Web.
40. Alban, Deane. "How to Balance Norepinephrine Levels Naturally." Be Brain Fit blog. 8 Jan 2019. Web.

41. Conger, Cristen. "Can you die of boredom?". How Stuff Works: Science blog. 6 May 2008. Web.

42. Winch, Guy. "The Important Difference Between Sadness and Depression... and why so many get it wrong." Psychology Today blog. 2 Oct 2015. Web.

43. Esposito, Linda. "The Surprising Emotion Behind Anxiety: Failing to recognize and express anger increases stress and health problems." Psychology Today blog. 25 Jul 206. Web.

44. Gautam, Medhavi; Agrawal, Mukta; Gautam, Manaswi; Sharma, Praveen; Sharma Gautam, Anita; Gautam, Shiv. " Role of antioxidants in generalised anxiety disorder and depression." US National Library of Medicine National Institutes of Health: Indian J Psychiatry. Jul-Sep 2012; 54(3): 244–247. Web.

References

45. Alexander, Katherine E.; Siegel, Harold I. "Perceived hunger mediates the relationship between attachment anxiety and emotional eating." Eating Behaviors: Volume 14, Issue 3, Pages 374-377. Aug 2013.

46. Davis, M.; Myers, K.M. "The role of glutamate and gamma-aminobutyric acid in fear extinction: clinical implications for exposure therapy." US National Library of Medicine National Institutes of Health: Biol Psychiatry. 15 Nov 2002; 15;52(10):998-1007.

47. Castro, Jason. "Scientists Gain Insights into How to Erase Pathological Fear." Scientific American blog. 14 Dec 2010. Web.

48. Macht, M. "Characteristics of Eating in Anger, Fear, Sadness and Joy." Institute for Psychology (I), University of Wu¨rzburg, Germany. Appetite: 1999, vol 33, 129–139 Article No. appe.1999.0236.

49. Macht, M. "Characteristics of Eating in Anger, Fear, Sadness and Joy." Institute for Psychology (I), University of Wu¨rzburg, Germany. Appetite: 1999, vol 33, 129–139 Article No. appe.1999.0236.

50. Bongers, P.; Jansen, A.; Havermans, R.; Roefs, A.; Houben,K.; Nederkoorn, C. "Happy eating. The role of positive mood in emotional eating." Appetite: Volume 71, Page 471. 1 Dec 2013.

51. Dubuc, Bruno. "How Drugs Affect Neurotransmitters." The Brain from Top to Bottom blog. 2002. Web.

52. Pychyl, Timothy. "How not to Be Pavlov's Dog:Individual differences in resisting temptation." Psychology Today blog. 24 Oct 2013. Web.

53. Neuroscientifically Challenged. "Know your brain: Reward system." 16 Jan 2015. Web.

www.ingramcontent.com/pod-product-compliance
Lightning Source LLC
Chambersburg PA
CBHW020615270326
41927CB00005B/345